NURSING HOME MINISTRY

Where Hidden Treasures Are Found

Bill Goodrich
&
Tom McCormick

God Cares Ministry

Copyright © 2003
God Cares Ministry

All rights reserved. No part of this book may be reproduced in any form, except for the inclusion of brief quotations in a review, without permission in writing from God Cares Ministry.

Library of Congress Card Number: pending

ISBN 0-9745384-0-X

Except when noted, all Scripture is taken from the HOLY BIBLE, NEW INTERNATIONAL VERSION. Copyright 1973, 1978, 1984 by the International Bible Society. Used by permission of the International Bible Society.

Several portions of text were taken, and used with permission, from Dr. Tom McCormick's Nursing Home Ministry – A Manual, which is now out of print.

Published by
God Cares Ministry
33399 Walker Rd., Suite A
Avon Lake, OH 44012
(440) 930-2173

Printed in the U.S.A. by Total Printing Systems

This book is dedicated to the
millions of people who will
finish life's journey
in a long-term care center.

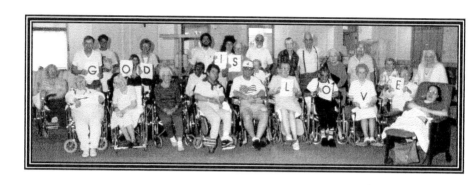

May the Lord continue to use them
to help His church experience
heaven's treasures.

John 15:9-13

TABLE OF CONTENTS

Changes 1

In the Beginning 3

Chapter 1   Introducing Nursing-Home Ministry 9
The Need 10
Nursing Homes in North America 12
You Are Needed in the Nursing Home 15
The Responsibility 18
Is Nursing Home Ministry My Calling? 22
Every Christians' Calling 24

Chapter 2   Preparing for Nursing-Home Ministry 26
Initial Preparations 27
Meeting the Activities Director 29
Further Preparations 31

**Chapter 3   What Every Nursing Home Missionary
              Needs to Know**................................. 34
You Can Have an Effective Nursing Home Ministry 36
The Spiritual Needs of Nursing Home Residents 39
Evangelism in the Nursing Home 47

Chapter 4   One-to-One Visiting 53
What is Visitation? 54
Guidelines for Visitation 55
What "To Be" 55
Guidelines for the First Few Visits 60
What to Say When You Don't Know What to Say 63

Chapter 5   Preparing A Way For The LORD 73
Rising Above Denominational Walls 74
Listening With Your Heart – Responding in Love 78
How To Lead A Resident To Jesus 82

Chapter 6   Care Teams and Group Services 89
The Ministry Care Team's Role 90
Worship Services 93
Suggested Model for Worship Services (Traditional) 94
Suggested Model for Worship Services (Casual) 96
Suggested Model For A Bible Study 98

Chapter 7   Tips for Effective Group Ministry 101
Some Guidelines for the Teacher 111
Three Parts of a Topical Sermon 114
Three Parts of a Bible Study 115
Group Ministry Evaluation 116

Chapter 8   Ministering Beyond the Limitations of Dementia 119
Perspectives on Dementia 124
Why Are We Uncomfortable? 125
Effective Ministry is Possible 126
Validation Ministry 129
Communication 132
The Ministry of the Word of God 136
A Bible Study That Breaks Through 137
We Minister by Faith and not by Sight 141
Tapping into Divine Power 143
Concerning Their Salvation 146

Chapter 9   Recruiting Help and Retaining It 150
Recruiting Your Pastor 152
Recruiting Church Members 156
Care Team Training 163
Keeping the Team Together 164
Nursing Home Ministry Seeds 166

v

Do's and Don'ts for Recruiting Volunteers 169

Chapter 10   Special Services and Activities 174
Communion Services 175
A Mobile Gospel Team 179
Residents in Ministry 180
Children and Youth in the Nursing Home 184
Resident Birthdays 190
Men's Woodshop 191
Opening Conversations with Pets 194
Special Outings 195
Conducting a Variety Show 198

Chapter 11   Special Issues and Concerns 201
Picture Taking 201
Receiving and Giving Gifts in the Nursing Home 203
Staff Relations 204
Other Special Concerns 207
What If You See Neglect or Abuse 210

Chapter 12   Ministering to the Grieving and the Dying . 215
Grief Defined 217
There Is a Good and Godly Grief 218
How Can I Help? 220
Ministering to the Dying 222
Funeral or Memorial Services 227

The Hidden Treasure 235

Acknowledgements 238

Resources and Resource People 240

Ordering Information 259

CHANGES

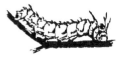

Nursing homes, assisted-living facilities, and adult family-care homes house primarily senior citizens who have once led productive lives. These seniors now need assistance from caregivers because their bodies or minds have become frail, and they are not able to keep up with the fast pace of society. That assistance ranges from basic housekeeping and meal preparation to extensive help with personal care, health issues and other activities of daily living.

Back in the 1980's, it was not uncommon in skilled-care nursing homes to find people who only needed basic assistance living among very frail seniors. Today, most people with only basic-care needs reside in assisted living facilities, allowing them much more independence. With the changes in health care, many seniors are being discharged from hospitals "quicker and sicker" and are often unable to remain in their homes. Therefore, the skilled-care nursing-home population has become more frail with more complex health care needs. Their need for spiritual care, however, is not so complex. In fact, nursing-home ministry is not just for professional clergy; many laypeople too are discovering the joy of this service and have become nursing-home missionaries.

The authors of this book realize the ongoing changes of the names and types of long-term care centers. We are also aware that titles of such facilities have changed over the years. Names and titles lose their social acceptance or meanings. In Elyria, Ohio, for example, there is a large multi-level care facility. When the home first opened up in 1896, it housed 25 women, and was called the "Old Ladies Home." Then, in 1923, it was re-named the "Home for the Aged" to include men. Then, "The Elyria

Methodist Home of the Northeast Ohio Conference of the Methodist Church" was adopted as residents objected to the word "aged;" now it is called "Elyria United Methodist Village." In time, the name will likely be changed yet again, as society changes its perspective or adopts different language.

Since the name "care center" is most commonly accepted for an overall title and the name "nursing home" is still commonly used throughout North America at the time of this writing, we have decided to use these terms interchangeably throughout the book. Our focus is primarily on the residents of nursing homes, because they are the most frail, needy, and neglected of long-term care residents. Of course, the teachings throughout this book can be, and have been, applied in all aspects of long-term care center ministry.

Though the names and duties of facilities housing senior citizens have changed over the years, the basic plight of residents in nursing homes has changed very little. For most, this is the final mile of their earthly journey. At this critical phase of life, much loving support is needed to help them find peace and hope for their future. Such a responsibility belongs to the church, and the Lord is calling many to embrace the responsibility of helping these dear people cross the finish line where they can receive the greatest treasure possible, a warm welcome from our God and Savior, Jesus Christ.

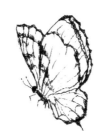

IN THE BEGINNING

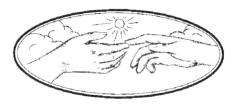

Bill & Mary Ann's story

Several years ago, my wife, Mary Ann, and I, began attending a fairly large church across town. Shortly after we became members, I received a call from the church secretary. She explained that she had heard we were involved in nursing home ministry and asked if we would visit Marjorie, a long-time member of the church. She explained that Marjorie was a very faithful servant of the Lord and had helped the church in many ways. Now she was in a nursing home and needed someone to be faithful to her.

A few days later, we made our first visit to the home where Marjorie was living. Although we had ministered and visited in other nursing homes, this home was different. It was much larger in size, but it also seemed to have a more depressing environment than other homes. Our impression, as we made our way to Marjorie's room, was that of a spiritual desert.

Hearing our knock, Marjorie turned toward us, smiled, and welcomed us in. She was a gracious woman who radiated peace and contentment. After a pleasant time of getting acquainted, I offered to read some Scriptures.

"What would you like me to read for you, Marjorie?" I asked. "Oh, I love the Psalms," she exclaimed. So for the next twenty minutes, I read several Psalms and we prayed for Marjorie. Then she prayed for us. What a beautiful time we all had! It was not at all difficult for us to return to visit Marjorie on almost a weekly basis.

After a few more visits, we learned that our new friend had cancer throughout her body. Once when I approached her open door and was getting ready to knock, I noticed Marjorie lying in her bed moaning, in obvious pain; she was turning her head back and forth and holding her stomach. Upon hearing our knock, Marjorie quickly composed herself as if nothing was wrong and welcomed us in. We again had a wonderful visit with Psalms and prayers, but we were now more aware of her agony. Before I left her room that day, I began to ask the Lord why He would allow such a beautiful child of His to experience so much suffering and pain. I received no immediate answer. It seemed as if God was silent.

As we made our way each week to and from Marjorie's room, we would pass a small chapel with stained glass windows, four pews, and some religious articles on an altar. I was often disturbed by the room's appearance because it was also being used to store wheelchairs, diapers, and extra lounge chairs. "What kind of place is this that they would build a sanctuary and then use it for storage?" I asked myself. In the five or six weeks we visited Marjorie, I never saw anyone in the chapel. One day after a visit with Marjorie, I entered the chapel and prayed, "Lord, this chapel is in a disgraceful condition. If you will make a way, I will start a Bible study in here."

After praying for a few days, I made an appointment to see the director of activities. In less than a week, my wife and I sat before this woman requesting permission to hold a weekly Bible study. She told us that she did not want any one coming in to evangelize or tell the residents they needed Jesus to be saved. After explaining our desire to share the Bible with any residents who desired to attend a weekly service, she cautiously agreed to give us a try, and the following Thursday we shared our first Bible study in that home. Seven residents and one very watchful activities assistant attended the service in the freshly-cleaned chapel. We shared the Word of God and the residents received it as if it were a cool drink of water in their desert.

Less than two weeks after we had begun the Bible study, the Lord took our dear friend Marjorie home to heaven. Although I was happy for her, I was also somewhat shocked. I went to the chapel and cried out to the Lord to help me understand the meaning of all these events. Within a few days, I began to realize that we were in the midst of God's perfect plan. Marjorie was the kind of servant who would say to the Lord, "Use me, Lord, I will do anything you want me to do." In my heart I believe the Lord had given Marjorie her final earthly mission. The people living in this nursing home needed the living water. The Lord wanted to use my wife and me to bring that water. Marjorie was the one God used to make us aware of the need and calling.

We met in the chapel for only three months; then we moved into a small dining room because the chapel was packed and the residents surrounding the doorway in the hall could not hear the entire message. About a year later, we had to move to the main lounge because it was the only space large enough for our growing group. Now, thirteen years later, we see how God has used us and other ministry team members to touch the lives of several hundred nursing-home residents who have finished life's journey in that home. We believe the Lord often sends people there that they may have one more chance to hear the Good News and be saved through His grace and the living Word of God, if they are not already Christians.

We are also involved in discipling Christians in the nursing home. Although the chapel is now too small for our weekly Bible studies, it is still used for a smaller group of residents. We meet almost weekly for an open discussion of Scripture, for prayer, and for coaching residents who are Christians in their outreach to new or bed-bound residents.

What started out as friendly visitation has led us deeper into one of the greatest mission fields in which the Lord has used us to help start or enhance hundreds of nursing-home ministry care teams. We look back now in awe as we realize it was the Lord asking for a drink through our dear sister Marjorie. By His grace, we responded, and have since experienced the promise He made to the Samaritan woman and every believer who will hear His call.

"If you knew the gift of God and who it is that asks you for a drink, you would have asked Him and He would have given you living water... Indeed, the

water I give him will become in him a spring of water welling up to eternal life." (John 4: 10, 14b)

Tom's story

The initiation I had to working in nursing homes is often a surprise to many. I had a lovely grandmother, but she was not a major influence in my life. Nor were there other older folk who could be "blamed" for my involvement with the elderly in nursing homes. I became involved in this type of ministry simply because I read the Bible and wanted to do what it said.

While I had grown up in church and never had any serious doubts about Jesus being the Way, I had not really been taught the Bible. After I graduated from the university, my conversion was not so much to Jesus, but to the Bible as God's own Word, with all wisdom and beauty, power and authority. Even though I was uncertain about many things, I simply decided to obey what was clear to me.

So I read the Bible, and in my reading I discovered the parable about the sheep and the goats in **Matthew 25**. This both scared me and touched my heart, for my family had always been sensitive to those in need. I also discovered *James 1:27*,

> *"Pure and undefiled religion in the sight of our God and Father is this: to visit orphans and widows in their distress, and to keep oneself unstained by the world." (NAS)*

This was clear to me and seemed to help me focus on what I should do. I didn't know of any orphans in my Indiana community, but I knew there were widows and other people with needs in nursing homes. I went to one home and asked if they had any jobs I could do. I was hired as a maintenance man, something I had experience doing. That, quite simply, is how my work in nursing homes began.

Shortly thereafter, I began Seminary training in Philadelphia. Not wanting to leave my newfound ministry with the elderly, I began work in nursing homes in the Philadelphia area. A retired professor who also had an interest in such work took me under his wing. Dr. John Skilton was to be my friend and companion and mentor for many years to come, in fact, until his death. He was a single man with a house to himself where he invited students to stay. I was privileged to live with him for several years, and it is there, at Skilton House (named after his beloved parents), that my work in nursing homes expanded and flourished.

As Dr. Skilton and I prayed, we decided to aim high. Our goal was to reach every resident in every nursing home in the Philadelphia area, including the surrounding suburbs. We began a several-year project of researching each home, charting needs in the homes, identifying churches close by, and offering to train local church people to reach the residents in nursing homes near them. Slowly, materials were developed as we conducted these sessions. Eventually a nursing home manual was published, initially by Great Commission Publications, and then by Zondervan.

We saw holidays as times of special need and opportunity in nursing homes. During the Christmas season and on both Good Friday and Easter, we planned city-wide efforts to reach every home and every resident in each home with a warm and personal Christian greeting and message. Seminary students and professors, lay people, and pastors all took part and we were largely successful year after year. We offered a special holiday service at those times annually, using each occasion to distribute large-print greeting cards which we mass-produced. We also developed large print greeting cards for other occasions, such as Valentine's Day and Thanksgiving. I still dream of developing a large-print greeting-card ministry.

From Philadelphia I began preparations for another phase of my life in mission work as a Bible translator and literacy worker in South America. Each step along the way of preparation for overseas work also provided further opportunity for work in nursing homes, this time in other states, including North Dakota and Texas. After returning from the mission field, I relocated to Toronto, Ontario, Canada, and began nursing-home work afresh. The ministry in Canada has given me a broader understanding of the situation in North America as a whole and the information in this training manual includes that broader perspective.

The rest of the story

Now Jesus had to go through Samaria. So he came to a town in Samaria called Sychar, near the plot of ground Jacob had given to his son Joseph. Jacob's well was there, and Jesus, tired as he was from the journey, sat down by the well. It was about the sixth hour. When a Samaritan woman came to draw water, Jesus said to her, "Will you give me a drink?" (John 4:6-8)

If Jesus asked you for a drink, what would you do? This woman did not know that it was Jesus, the Messiah, asking her for a drink. To the woman, Jesus was only a man, specifically, in fact, a man who was of a race that traditionally looked down on her own people. But Jesus said to her, *"If you knew the gift of God and who it is that asks you for a drink..." (John 4:9)*. If she had only known it was Jesus! If she had only known that for her to give this stranger a drink, it would have been remembered for all eternity! If she had only known the great privilege and opportunity that God was offering her and what a blessing it would be for her!

There are thousands of people in our communities who do not even have the ability to ask us for a drink because they are hidden behind the walls of long-term care centers, commonly called nursing homes. They are some of the loneliest people in our society. Yet these people have also become the best of friends to many who have taken steps of faith to share God's love and Word with them.

We invite you to take a step of faith by studying the Scriptures and principles in this book and applying them in care centers in your church's community. We are sure that as you engage in ministry, the Lord will richly bless you with some of heaven's eternal treasures.

CHAPTER 1

INTRODUCING NURSING-HOME MINISTRY

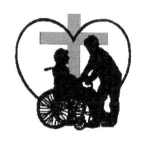

In those days, when the number of disciples was increasing, the Grecian Jews among them complained against the Hebraic Jews because their widows were being overlooked in the daily distribution of food. So the Twelve gathered all the disciples together and said, "It would not be right for us to neglect the ministry of the Word of God in order to wait on tables. Brothers, choose seven men from among you who are known to be full of the Spirit and wisdom. We will turn this responsibility over to them and will give our attention to prayer and the ministry of the Word." This proposal pleased the whole group. They chose Stephen, a man full of faith and of the Holy Spirit; also Philip, Procorus, Nicanor, Timon, Parmenas, and Nicolas from Antioch, a convert to Judaism. They presented these men to the apostles, who prayed and laid their hands on them. <u>So the Word of God spread</u>. The number of disciples in Jerusalem increased rapidly, and a large number of priests became obedient to the faith (Acts 6:1-7).

Sometimes growth starts with recognizing the true needs of those around us. In **Acts 6:1-7**, we see our church fathers were presented with a need. Their response to that need resulted in advancing the kingdom of God. The need for the early church was to minister to the widows; as a result, the widows were blessed, but so were many others.

THE NEED

In *those* days, during a great movement of the Lord, the widows were being overlooked. In *these* days, there is still a tendency in the church to overlook and even shy away from the responsibility of caring for the widows and elderly, particularly those confined to long-term care centers like nursing homes. Unfortunately, this frail population may even be considered a burden because they consume resources, time, and energy, and may appear to give little if anything in return. Yet in **1 Corinthians 12:21-25,** God said,

> *"The eye cannot say to the hand, 'I don't need you!' And the head cannot say to the feet, 'I don't need you!' On the contrary, those parts of the body that seem to be weaker are indispensable... ...There should be no division in the body, but that its parts should have equal concern for each other."*

The truth is, as the body of Christ, we who are strong and vibrant need those people who are older and frailer every bit as much as they need us. The best way for those of us who are able-bodied to understand the need we have for frail seniors is to spend quality time in nursing-home ministry. The residents who live in nursing homes, will soon become an important part of our lives as we faithfully visit. Indeed, God will use the relationships that are established to teach us more about the true meaning of Christ-like love. In knowing, serving, and loving people in need, we also come to know, serve and love our Lord Jesus Christ more intimately. **(Matthew 25:40).**

The primary reason people move into nursing homes is related to personal health problems and their inability to care for themselves or be cared for at home. It is a rare occasion to hear a resident say that he[1] preferred living in the nursing home rather than his own home. The following quote conveys this point:

> *"Most of the residents have lost the things on this earth that are dearest to them: their mate, their home, and either their finances or the control over them. The average residents are people who, with their mates, once made all their own decisions: where to live, when and what to eat, what to wear, where to go, how to spend their time, and money, etc. Suddenly, and in many cases in only a short period of time, almost all their decisions and choices are taken from them. Now they are told when to eat, when to go to bed, when to get up, what to wear, etc. Some people adjust better than others, but it is a traumatic experience for all. In most cases there is rebellion, either outward or inward or both. Regardless, they must learn to cope with and exist with it. They are without any real choice in the matter."*
>
> *Herm Haakenson, All The Days of My Life*

Nursing-home residents have many physical and social needs. Most nursing homes strive to provide a high-quality physical and social atmosphere that is as pleasant as possible. However, even with the best physical and social care, there may be unmet spiritual needs, including the need to prepare for death. Residents often have unresolved conflicts and unanswered

---

[1] To save room and maintain free flow, we decided to use the pronouns, "him, his, he" rather than "him/her etc."

questions that living in an institution seems to magnify. It is not uncommon to hear questions and comments like, "Does God really care about me?" "God must be punishing me." "I wish that God would take me home now." "I never thought I would end up in a place like this." "Where is my family now?" "My pastor has only visited me one time in over two years." "I used to go to church, but I don't go any more." These needs and concerns are generally accompanied with fear, disappointment, despair, and even hopelessness.

Though there is nothing that can be done to stop the aging process itself, Much *can* be done to strengthen or restore the soul of even the most physically and/or mentally challenged person.

> *"Though outwardly we are wasting away, yet inwardly we are being renewed, day by day."*
>
> **2 Corinthians 4:16**

NURSING HOMES IN NORTH AMERICA

In the United States and Canada there are over 20,000 nursing homes, ranging in size from six beds to sometimes over three hundred, with the average size being just over 100 beds per home. The smaller homes, as you might imagine, can provide a more family-like, intimate atmosphere, while the larger homes are like a small community within a community.

Currently there are approximately 2 million people living in nursing homes in the United States and Canada combined. The need for nursing-home beds is expected to at least double by the year 2025 to keep pace with the aging baby-boomer generation.

> **Did You Know...?**
>
> *Over 90% of nursing home residents are age 65+*
> *They are 5% of USA's 65+ population*
> *and 8% of Canada's 65+ population.*
>
> *Over 50% of nursing home residents are age 85+*
> *They are 24% of USA's 85+ population*
> *and 40% of Canada's 85+ population.*

The people who live in nursing homes come from every walk of life. Many were poor and many were affluent; many lived ethical and productive lives and many did not. About two-thirds of all nursing-home residents are women, who generally live longer than men. The average age of women in nursing homes is about eighty-three years; the average age of men is seventy-six. It is estimated that more then 50,000,000 people now living in North America will spend their last days in one type of long-term care facility. This includes people of all different nationalities and ethnic backgrounds.

There are many types of long-term care facilities such as assisted living, adult family homes, and congregate living facilities; though nursing homes are the most common venue for church outreach. Each type of facility provides services to assist their residents with what are called "activities of daily living" (ADLs).

> **Did You Know...?**
>
> *97% of nursing home residents require help with ADL's such as bathing, dressing, eating, transfer from bed to chair, and the use of the toilet.*
> *75% need help with 3 or more ADLs.*

Nursing homes are required by regulatory agencies to provide spiritual care for their residents. Staff members who are

Christians often do this individually, by praying for residents, for example, but their time is very limited. Some nursing homes have a spiritual care director or a chaplain on staff to minister to the residents' spiritual needs. Regardless, the nursing homes rely heavily on local churches to assist them with worship services, Bible studies, pastoral and friendly visitation. To the shame of the church, some activities directors have testified they were not able to find a church in the community willing to help assist in providing spiritual care on a regular basis. It is the purpose of this book to help remedy that situation.

> *Our care-team coordinator, Lucy, asked me if I could play piano for the nursing-home ministry, I didn't feel I could refuse, for after all, I do play piano. And I make my own work schedule. Still I wasn't really sure that it was something I wanted to do. After all, who really wants to go to a nursing home? I thought about it and prayed about it and I decided that if all she wanted me to do was play piano, I could do that.*
>
> *A normal visit for me included helping set up microphones and then playing jazz standards on the piano as others wheel in the residents. Then I'd play hymns during our service. I was comfortable with that.*
>
> *But my visit to the nursing home was different for me today. Lucy, (organized person that she is) got there early. Not only did she set everything up, but she also put on a CD for the time before the service. My crutch was gone! I didn't have anything to do! What would I do? What do I have to say to these people?!*
>
> *When Lucy went to bring residents in, I tagged along with her. "Hi John." " How are you, Mary?" She said sweetly. Lucy seems so natural with the residents. Soon I noticed how she started some conversations. Maybe it isn't so hard! Just look around at what the people are*

doing! After a few minutes, I struck out on my own. Maybe I could talk to a few people, too.

As I did, I noticed how the residents changed when I spoke with them. One bent woman attended our services regularly, but I'd never met her yet. From the blank look on her face I wondered if she'd even know what I was saying when I introduced myself. As soon as I spoke, she sat up a smidge taller in her wheelchair. A light seemed to spark in her eyes. Her agonizingly slow words revealed an intelligent, fun-loving person. Soon Trudy and I were laughing together.

No, I didn't lead anyone to Christ today. But through Him I was able to step out of my comfort zone and fellowship with another of His sheep. I still don't feel completely comfortable at the nursing home. But I do feel like that this is where God wants me.

What comfort zone is Christ challenging you to step out of today?

Dawn Purney

YOU ARE NEEDED IN THE NURSING HOME

The needs of residents in nursing homes and the opportunities to minister to them are vast and varied. Here we share some of the reasons Christian volunteers are needed:

The staff needs you:

Nursing-home personnel are responsible for the well being of the residents, including, but not limited to, providing a clean and safe home, nutritious meals, personal hygiene, and medical assistance, along with recreational, social, and spiritual activities. Nursing-home staff are also required to comply with very tough certification and licensing regulations. The pay rate for nursing assistants, those who work closest to the residents, is generally low, resulting in a high turnover rate. Staff members appreciate volunteers who have a genuine concern for and interest in each resident's well-being. They realize you are meeting an **important** need when you are able to spend quality time with the residents. A humble and courteous attitude to all staff will open many doors that might otherwise have remained closed. Such an attitude will help you to be seen as a blessing, and not as a burden. In time, you will become more familiar with staff members, giving you opportunities to befriend and bless them personally as well.

> Although nursing home's are required to offer spiritual care for each resident, it is the responsibility of churches to provide it.

The residents need you:

Residents will often experience a phase of cultural shock upon entering a care center. They face the challenge of being a stranger in an extremely different environment than they are used to living. They often struggle with the stereotypes of *"old folks in the nursing home"*. These and other concerns can be the cause of fear, grief, depression, anger, etc., leading to a "survival behavior" uncharacteristic of their former mannerism.

Loneliness is another pain that can best be relieved by being with others who care. Many residents have simply outlived most of their friends and relatives; friends and relatives who are still living may rarely visit. Many feel that their relatives and churches have actually abandoned them. Therefore, one of the greatest things we can do is just be there for them.

> **Culture shock** *is the sense of cultural disorientation one experiences while living in a different society from his own. It carries with it:*
> - *emotional anxiety from being in strange surroundings*
> - *disorientation from not being able to predict what other people are going to do.*
> - *discomfort from not knowing how to handle unfamiliar situations.*

Visitation is our privilege and can often provide opportunities to help residents put their hope and trust in Christ! Many residents do not understand that they can have a **personal** relationship with Jesus and that He can meet all their needs. They may have misunderstandings and/or concerns about religion, which they would talk about if someone they trusted would take the time to listen. Residents who are already Christians may or may not have a strong relationship with the Lord. They, too, need encouragement through the love and Word of God and support in being active in their faith.

> *To love and be loved gives a person purpose and hope for tomorrow. When these are missing, many find no reason for living.*

The families need you:

Family members have often told us they were greatly comforted knowing that someone is spending time with their loved one. Sometimes a resident will openly share things with a trusted friend that he would not share with a family member. In ministering to people living in nursing homes, we are encouraged to not become personally involved with family conflicts or giving medical and financial advise, as these normally create unnecessary problems. However, our willingness to listen and respectfully share in prayer can become the bridge to God's peace. We have had the opportunity to attend numerous funerals to comfort the family and assure them of their loved one's personal and present relationship with Jesus.

God needs you:

It is true that the Lord can do whatever He desires without us. However, His divine plan is to do much of His great work through His disciples. Every person who was led to Jesus, was led through the efforts of other Christians who were being used by God directly or indirectly. Serving the King of Kings is not only our responsibility; it is a great privilege. As Mother Theresa often said, "We are His hands and feet".

THE RESPONSIBILITY

Not every individual Christian is called into nursing-home ministry, but every church should have a vision to serve in at least one long-term care center in their community. The responsibility that Christians have to provide quality spiritual care in care centers can be divided into two areas. The first is the responsibility of the individual who feels called to this ministry, and the second is the responsibility of the church.

Individual Responsibility

Wherever we turn in the Bible, we consistently see exhortations to **honor** the aged and the widow. In the Ten Commandments, (**Exodus 20:1-17**) we find the well-known commandment to honor fathers and mothers, whatever their age. Other commandments prohibit afflicting or taking advantage of the widow (for example, **Exodus 22:22**). **Proverbs 23:22** says, **"Listen to your father who gave you life, and do not despise your mother when she is old."** Leviticus 19:32 also makes our attitude to the elderly abundantly clear: **"You shall rise up before the grayheaded, and honor the aged...."** The New Testament likewise promotes an attitude of honor as it reiterates the command to honor parents, in particular (**Matthew 15:1-9; Ephesians 6:2-3**) and the elderly, in general (**I Timothy 5:1-3**).

The scriptural examples of honor and dishonor give us a clear idea of exactly what honor is. In relation to honoring God through sacrifice and through his Son **(Malachi 1:6-14; 1Samuel 2:29-30; John 5:22-23)**, we see that to honor is to esteem, revere, regard, respect, give recognition to, or recognize the value, importance, or significance of someone. The opposite of honoring would be to despise, reject, mock, show contempt for, be ashamed of, or speak evil of someone **(Isaiah 53:3; Psalm 22:6, 7; Deuteronomy 28:49, 50; Proverbs 30:17; Matthew 15:1-9)**. Unfortunately, the latter has often found expression in our culture, especially in respect to the aged.

Another responsibility we have is to protect the aged and the widow. **Isaiah 1:16-17** tells us to plead the case of the widow. And **1Timothy 5:3-16** urges us to take care of widows and warns us about neglecting them.

Consider the situation that a widow is in. She has lost her spouse who was a protector and a trustworthy friend who normally helped carry the load of responsibility and decision making around the home. When this support is taken away, widows are left in a vulnerable and sometimes overwhelming condition. And, unfortunately, they are often neglected or taken advantage of by greedy and inconsiderate people offering them deals they "cannot refuse". Christians do well to build relationships with close neighbor widows, offering help with areas in which they are struggling. Help can also be given to widows (and widowers) in nursing homes, especially those who may also be childless or have children who may not visit frequently.

Sometimes we think we have so little to offer, but I was taught differently a few weeks ago. I was walking down the hall of a nursing home and a resident who was using a walker and moving very slow realized I had come up behind her so she stopped and said, "That's OK, just go around." I just wanted to walk with her so I paused for a moment and said, "I'm in no hurry." Again, she motioned and said, "Go ahead", but I said, "I prefer to walk with you if that's OK." So we walked along and talked for a few minutes. As we approached the end of our short journey she said, "Thank you so much for taking the time to be with me. Everyone is in such a hurry around here." I thought to myself of how much the little effort I made had meant so much to her. Then I realized that just a little time and kindness shared with those who are lonely becomes a very meaningful treasure to them.
Shared by a care-team member at a training workshop.

Any Christian with a caring heart for those living in care centers can make an eternal difference by following the basic guidelines outlined in this book and using the resources available. Special talents or education can be helpful but they are not a prerequisite. Many individuals have started a viable nursing home ministry simply by just committing to visit one or two residents on a regular basis.

The Christian Visitor

...is a Bible believer who has received Christ as personal Savior;
...is Christ-like and thus has a heart of love, care, compassion and concern for others;
...takes time in prayer and in the Word to prepare for each visit;
...is regular in visiting, as a testimony to the Lord's faithfulness.

Tom and Kaye DePinto, Nursing Home Ministry

Responsibility of the Church

Churches have a responsibility to people living in long-term care centers too. The church can honor and protect by recognizing nursing-home ministry as a local-mission field. Since there is a care center in almost every community, we do not need to move missionary teams to another country. Nonetheless, we must keep in mind that this small community within our community is a mission field and is of no less importance than any mission field overseas.

> **Did You Know...?**
> Some foreign missionaries give their entire productive lives to working with people groups less than the size of most nursing homes.

When the church continually neglects training, equipping, sending and supporting missionaries for serving in nursing homes, it is neglecting a primary calling. There are several Scriptures that validate this point, but there is none as clear as *James 1:27:*

> ***Religion that God our Father accepts as pure and faultless is this: to look after orphans and widows in their distress and to keep oneself from being polluted by the world.***

With a word so clear, how is it that we have missed the mark? Churches outnumber long-term care centers more than eight to one, and yet there are still too many residents who do not receive adequate spiritual care. Some homes have chaplains on staff but many more do not and rely solely on volunteer church involvement.

Many nursing-home residents fear their future because they do not personally know the Good Shepherd. Many are craving the Bread of Life and thirsting for the Living Water. The responsibility to help meet these and other spiritual needs of nursing-home residents may seem overwhelming, but consider: if *each church* in America would *establish only one care team* and *adopt only <u>one</u> nursing-home*, the spiritual needs of the residents in every nursing home could be met. It is a very simple solution; the primary requirement is commitment. Thankfully, many churches have responded to the call but many more have not. There is still an urgency to blow the trumpet and sound the alarm until the need is fully met.

IS NURSING HOME MINISTRY MY CALLING?

Sometimes, as Christians, we may wonder what God's will is for our lives and what kind of Christian service we are supposed to be involved in. We can and should know God's basic calling for our lives.

> **"Delight yourself in the Lord and he will give you the desire of your heart."**
> **Psalm 37:4**

Sometimes God calls His people in very special ways. For instance, in **Acts 9:10-18,** God called Ananias in a vision, giving him a specific task, of going to a specific place, to fulfill a specific purpose. Many of the characters in the Bible have received this *specific* kind of calling. Although we may desire such a vision, it is not the most common method the Lord uses to send workers into His harvest field.

The other more usual kind of calling is found in Scriptures like *Matthew 25:31-40, Isaiah 58:6-12* and *James 1:27.* These and many other Scriptures are quite clear that all Christians are called to serve those less fortunate, but the particulars are not usually specified. We therefore have the liberty to choose the specific type of ministry where we sense the greatest need. The important issue is not to bury any of our gifts for serving others, but rather to use them in practical and loving ways that honor and glorify the Lord.

> **He guides me in paths of righteousness
> for His name's sake.**
>
> **Psalm 23:3**

With this in mind you may ask, "What areas have the greatest needs?" and "How can my life be most fruitful?" As noted, people confined to institutions such as nursing homes are among those most greatly deprived of quality Christ-centered spiritual care. Some of the reasons for this deprivation are:

- Nursing-home residents are not able to search for a church to help meet their spiritual needs. Instead, they have to wait for the church to come to them. If a church group comes into a home or the home is fortunate enough to have a chaplain, residents are able to attend church, though not necessarily a church of their own choosing.

- Members of a local church may come to the nursing home but not take the privilege seriously enough to provide a quality service.

- There may or may not be a consistent Bible studies and personal visits, depending on the commitment of the church or individual Christians.

> **Jesus said, "I tell you, open your eyes and look at the fields! They are ripe for harvest!"**
>
> **John 4:35**

EVERY CHRISTIAN'S CALLING

Returning to **(Acts 6:1-7)**; we see that the Apostles took care of the problem of the neglected widows by choosing a small group of people to meet their needs. Those chosen were known to be full of the Spirit and wisdom. Fullness of the Spirit and wisdom comes from God Himself. He gives His Spirit to those who love Jesus and obey His commands, **(John 14:15-21)** and His wisdom is given to those who ask in faith without doubting **(James 1:2-8)**. Clearly, there are many ministry needs in every community, and God is calling all Christians to join Him in meeting these needs. However, He is first calling us to our Lord Jesus Himself. Abiding in Jesus is our primary calling. As we abide (or remain) in Jesus, He will abide in us; then we will **know** God's will and have the ability to walk in His power. Although nursing-home ministry is a field in which all Christians can labor, our fruitfulness depends on our faithfulness to abiding in our Lord Jesus and His Word.

> *Jesus said, "I am the vine; you are the branches. If a man remains in me and I in him, he will bear much fruit; apart from me you can do nothing." (John 15:5)*

Is our Lord calling you to further involvement in this mission field? Will you prayerfully consider that possibility? The following chapters will give you more information about long-term care centers and the people you could be serving. You will also be given many resources to help you share the love and Word of God in the nursing home He might be calling you in to minister.

It does not take many visits to a nursing home before one discovers that by God's grace, we all have the great treasure of **time** to share with the very people who become our treasured friends. The closer we are to Jesus, the more abundantly we can give; not only time, but love and the Word of life. And it truly is in giving that we will also receive.

"Give, and it will be given to you. A good measure, pressed down, shaken together and running over, will be poured into your lap. For with the measure you use, it will be measured to you." (Luke 6:38)

Then I heard the voice of the Lord saying, "Whom shall I send? And who will go for us?" And I said, "Here am I. Send me!" (Isaiah 6:8)

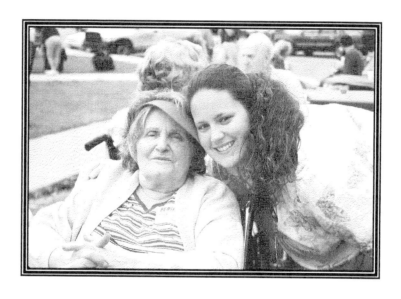

Dear friends, let us love one another, for love comes from God. Everyone who loves has been born of God and knows God.

1John 4:7

CHAPTER 2

PREPARING FOR NURSING-HOME MINISTRY

A few months after taking a Nursing Home Ministry Training Class, I took my mother-in-law to a senior citizens' luncheon at a local church. Noticing a young woman helping several older men with their lunch, I asked if they were from a nursing home. When it was affirmed that they were, I asked if the nursing home might like to have a weekly Bible Study. The woman said, "Yes, I'm sure we would," and gave the name and phone number of the Activities Director. When I called and shared what we wanted to do, she almost cried. She had been praying for someone to do just what we were offering.

Bernice Schaefer

Over the past several years, we have had the privilege of helping many churches start or enhance a nursing-home ministry care team. A care team is a small group of people committed to work together to share the love and Word of Jesus through one-to-one visits and/or group worship services and Bible studies. It only takes two people to make a team for one-to-one visiting. For group worship services, a team of four or more is usually recommended. (See Chapter 6 for a detailed description of a care team for worship services.)

INITIAL PREPARATIONS

Starting a nursing-home ministry care team in your church may seem an overwhelming task to plan and implement. But it is precisely good planning that will help make your ministry effective and less overwhelming. We recommend the following initial steps be taken:

> **Commit your works to the Lord and your plans will be established.**
>
> **Proverbs 16:3**

1. **Pray:** Pray especially for wisdom, understanding, and direction. A season of prayer and fasting has been the practice of many believers who have experienced the Lord's presence in their ministry. Many of us have made unnecessary mistakes because we have not taken the time to pray. If possible, pray with other believers who are currently ministering in a nursing home.

2. **Study God's Word:** It is important to understand God's perspective on any ministry if we desire to be effective. In this book you will find over one hundred Scripture references related to this ministry and the Bible has many more.

3. **Seek to obtain Pastoral support:** It is your pastor's responsibility to help equip you and facilitate lay ministry in the church **(Ephesians 4:11-12)**. Your pastor needs to have confidence that you will conduct yourself in a manner worthy of the gospel of Christ **(Philippians 1:27)**. Ask him to pray for you and to encourage other church members to team up with you in either ministry or

intercessory prayer. This kind of pastoral support will be most helpful and encouraging to all the team members.

4. **Recruit volunteers:** Find out if there is anyone in your church currently visiting in a nursing home. Seek to build a team together. It is important to be organized when you recruit. Remember, when recruiting help, you are asking people to give one of life's most valued resources: time. Volunteers need to sense that there is a viable need and a specific plan to meet the need. It is a good idea to welcome creative suggestions in the planning stages, though you may also need to "prime the pump" with concrete possibilities. Pray together that God will guide you in these important decisions. Be prepared to adjust your plans as you become more familiar with the nursing home and the individuals with whom you come in contact there.

5. **Decide on a nursing home:** Often a church will look for a nursing home in their community and find that there are several within a twenty-minute drive. Wanting to have the most impact, they choose to divide their time between four or five homes, visiting each home once a month, on a rotating basis. Although this may sound like a good idea, we highly recommend that you choose **only one** home that is very near to your church. There are a number of reasons for this:

- The closer the nursing home is to the church, the more accessible it will be for most church members.

- After you are well established and effectively ministering in the home, your faithfulness will be a testimony to your community. **(John 13:35)**

- The closer your church is to the nursing home, the more accessible it will be for residents and/or staff who may want to attend.

- Weekly visits in one home enable you to establish deeper relationships with residents, staff, and family. The better we know our friends, the more we understand their needs and how to help them.

- Teams that rotate on a monthly basis take more effort to organize and maintain.

> We do not want to give the impression that once-a-month visits are inappropriate. They can be a great blessing! But, please keep these points in mind while planning your outreach.

When a church has the ability to have more than one care team, it is prudent to have the other teams minister in other homes. We also recommend that these teams all be overseen under one leader, but that they work independently of each other.

If you have several options for appropriately located homes, visit each one, investigate the possibilities in each place, pray, discuss and make a decision as a team. (Chapters 9 & 10 have more details about recruiting and planning your programs.)

MEET WITH THE ACTIVITIES DIRECTOR

Nursing homes are normally in great need of volunteers and will welcome your church's participation. They may, however, enforce certain restrictions and limitations because they do not know you. They may also require you to attend orientation or training sessions. Always be submissive and respectful. In time, you will build a trusting relationship. Normally, the activities director of the nursing home will be your primary contact. This is the person with whom you want to make an appointment to meet and share your desires. If the home has a chaplain or volunteer coordinator, you may be directed to one of them.

Your opening statement when you call the activities director can be, "Hello. I am ___ from ___ church. I would like to know if you would be interested in some of our members volunteering to visit residents at your facility?" If you are asked what it is you specifically want to do, you can say, "We would like to establish friendships with some of your residents who would appreciate a friendly visitor" and/or "We would like to conduct worship services, Bible studies, etc." If there is any hesitation from the activities director, it is likely related to a concern that you would be proselytizing. If this concern is brought up, you may want to say, "Our purpose is not to try to change people's religion, but we would like to read the Bible and pray for those who desire it."

If the activities director is interested, he will likely invite you for an interview and a tour of the facility. Try to involve as many team members as are available to go with you. Whether or not all team members can go, the team leader should be prepared, appropriately dressed, and on time.

> Don't be apprehensive about this meeting. You can be fairly certain that the activities director is excited about finding trustworthy volunteers to help with activities and personal visits.

When you meet with the activities director, you will want to give a clear and concise overview of your desires. He will want to know what church you represent, your pastor's name, and the primary contact person to call if there are any questions or concerns. It is not uncommon for a care center to require a background check (including fingerprinting) and a tuberculosis (TB) test. This is done to safeguard the residents and should be complied with.

Once the required information is shared, the activities director will work out an agreeable schedule and give you a list of residents to visit and/or help you choose a group activity that is appropriate to the needs of the home and your interests. If your desire is to start a Bible study or church service, we recommend that you first spend a month or two visiting one-to-one. This will not only enable you to build a rapport with the residents and staff, it will help you become more acquainted and comfortable with the nursing-home environment. It is also a good idea to have the activities director introduce you to some of the key staff people in the home and for you to be known by them. Of course, you will also want to be introduced to the residents on the list. As time progresses, you will have an accepted, and hopefully, valued place in the life of the home. Be prepared to begin a ministry slowly and, by your words and deeds, earn the right to freely minister in the home.

FURTHER PREPARATIONS

Again, *prayer* is essential for your effectiveness. A few other things will also help prepare you and your team members:

- **Training:** We recommend that you provide some basic training. This can be done through sharing portions of this book, showing a nursing home-ministry training video (see our Resource Chapter), or inviting other, experienced ministry-team members in your area to share their insights. You may also want to invite the activities director to communicate basic principles and nursing-home policies. Whatever the approach to training you choose, hold on to this appreciated rule, **"Keep It Simple."**

- **Resources:** Present any resources available for effective nursing-home ministry. One of the largest producers of such resources is the Sonshine Society of Lynnwood, WA. See our Resource Chapter for a complete listing of their products.

- **Learn:** Your understanding of aging, long-term care centers, and the place of suffering in human life will help you be more effective in your outreach.

- **Communicate:** Write out the chosen schedule and brief details to prevent any miscommunication among the team members.

- **Prepare a "log book":** Some have used a log book to record specific information like prayer requests, promises made, special needs, etc. This could help facilitate future visits/contacts.

- **Be strong and courageous:** Trust that you can do all things through Christ who gives you strength. **(Joshua 1:9)**

Beginning a nursing-home ministry in your church is not difficult. It is like gardening; it takes some planning, preparing, sowing and maintaining. Many of the seeds you sow will be merely tiny seeds of faith and obedience. At times, these seeds may seem insignificant; but remember what Jesus said the kingdom of God is like:

"It is like a mustard seed, which is the smallest seed you plant in the ground. Yet when planted, it grows and becomes the largest of all garden plants, with such big branches that the birds of the air can perch in its shade" (Mark 4:31-32).

Like a mustard seed, a ministry care team planted in a nursing home will grow to become a great source of comfort for many.

One candle can light a thousand candles if the part that carries the light can touch the part that can receive the light. By faith, our hearts can carry the Light of the world into dark places and the glory of the Lord will rise!

For God, who said, "Let light shine out of darkness," made his light shine in our hearts to give us the light of the knowledge of the glory of God in the face of Christ. But we have this treasure in jars of clay to show that this all-surpassing power is from God and not from us.

2 Corinthians 4:6-7

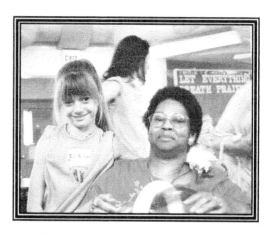

The people living in darkness have seen a great light; on those living in the land of the shadow of death a light has dawned (Matthew 4:16).

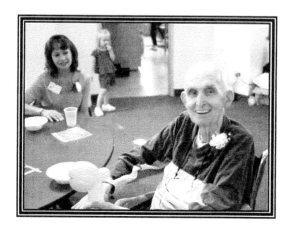

CHAPTER 3

WHAT EVERY NURSING HOME MISSIONARY NEEDS TO KNOW

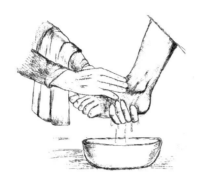

Several months ago we met a dear woman who was no longer eating and was unresponsive to medical treatment. Mary's words to us were, "I feel like I'm dying inside." The story that began to unfold as we gained her trust was the story of one who had literally been "cast off in (her) old age," and "forsaken when (her) strength had failed" **(Psalm 71:9).**

The past year had brought unimaginable heartbreak to this 75-year-old woman. Her husband of fifty-four years died suddenly of a heart attack. Shortly before his death, their daughter and granddaughter were tragically killed in a car accident. Then, not long after her husband's death, Mary suffered a severe stroke that required three months of rehabilitation in a care center. It was during this time, without her knowledge or consent, that her son sold the home she had lived in for forty-five years in the little town where all her friends lived, and then made arrangements to have his mother moved into the nursing home. The deepest wound of all, however, was that her son left her in the nursing home without even saying good-bye.

Needless to say, these events had taken a dreadful toll on Mary. She had trusted in Jesus Christ as her Savior when she was a child, and had followed Him faithfully through the years; but now, weak, grieving, and utterly alone, her pain was more than she could bear. She began to withdraw into a long, lonely winter of despair.

We visited Mary week after week. We spent time with her, listened to her, prayed with her, and read the Word together with her. Then we watched in wonder as God's grace accomplished a work of transformation in her life. Mary's faith in the Lord began to blossom again and grow stronger each day as He brought comfort and healing to her heart. The seasons in her life were beginning to change as Mary's faith in Jesus, the Resurrection and the Life, was rekindled.

During our most recent visit with Mary, her roommate, Doris, overheard our conversation. Doris was touched by Mary's praise to God for His continued faithfulness in the midst of her trials and tears. As she listened attentively to the story of Mary's miraculous metamorphosis from despair to hope, she wanted to hear more about Jesus. Through God's Word, Mary's testimony and our prayers, the Holy Spirit ministered to her, and Doris trusted in Jesus as her personal Savior that day.

Chaplain Stacy Waller,
Love Your Neighbor Ministries

YOU CAN HAVE AN EFFECTIVE NURSING-HOME MINISTRY

If you were to go to another country as a missionary, you would need to study and adjust to the people's language and culture in which they live. The people living in nursing homes are from a different generation then most of us and have a language and culture that is unique. Ministry includes being sensitive to their traditions and rituals in which they are accustomed. As with the Apostle Paul, we need to adapt and become all things to all people so that by all possible means we might save some **(1 Corinthians 9:22)**. The following four points should also be considered for effective visitation ministry:

1. Nursing-home ministry is different from other ministries.

All people have the same basic spiritual needs. However, the **method** of addressing and helping people obtain fulfillment of these needs is different according to their special circumstances and background. If we try to approach nursing-home ministry the same way we might approach other ministries, such as street evangelism or prison ministry, we will certainly experience problems. In fact, one of the primary reasons for frustration in nursing-home ministry is a failure to understand how to reach out appropriately to residents. Nursing-home ministry is a specialized mission field where any Christian who loves the Lord and people can bear much fruit. However, the more we understand about aging, long-term care centers, and what experienced nursing-home missionaries have learned throughout the years, the more effective we will become.

It is also important to understand issues and experiences that can result from the resident's mental or physical frailties.

> *Once a lady named Agnes, who had mild dementia told me (Bill) that her roommate had men visiting her at night and she whispered, "I wouldn't want to tell you some of the things they say and do." Agnes told me that I should stay away from her. I thought for a long time, "She is fairly cognizant. Why would she say that? I know it cannot be true." Later on, I did meet her roommate. After some conversation, she told me that she has a hard time sleeping at night because of her breathing problems. She explained that she watched the late-night movies that were sometimes not fit for television. "But I can't sleep and that's all that's on," she told me. I finally realized that these were the voices Agnes heard on the other side of the curtain.*

Had I hastily tried to fix this above "problem", I might have caused a considerable amount of trouble. Nursing-home missionaries need to realize that in any established environment, there are certain unwritten manners and styles of being that can only be learned and understood through time and by quiet observation.

2. We must respect care centers' policies and procedures.

All nursing homes must pass state and federal surveys in order to maintain their license and receive needed financial reimbursements. Regulatory criteria for nursing homes include many policies and procedures. For example: visitors and staff should respect the privacy of residents and knock before entering a resident's room. In general, visitors should not take it upon themselves to transfer a resident from a bed to a chair or feed a resident; both of these rules relate to issues of safety. There may also be some not-so-obvious policies that could sometimes appear odd or even inappropriate. We must realize that we are under the authority of the care-center staff and it is our responsibility to submit to them and abide by the rules of the home

(Romans 13:1-5). If a certain rule seems to be unfitting, we do well to respectfully seek a better understanding of its purpose.

3. We must leave our denomination at our church.

There are many denominations represented in a nursing home. We must be careful to respect the residents and the freedom they have to believe and practice according to their traditions. We must also be sensitive to not offend other Christians by our own denominational practices. The role of worship is to help people call upon the name of the Lord Jesus. Residents who are open to the Christian faith appreciate a service in which Jesus is lifted up (without any denominational dogma). Once they are in Jesus' care, He will move any *straying believers* to worship the Father in Spirit and truth. We will cover this topic in more detail. See Rising Above Denominational Walls" in chapter 5.

> *"Everyone who calls on the name of the Lord will be saved."*
>
> **Acts 2:21**

4. We must love the people we serve, and pray for them.

Prayer is essential to effective ministry. Someone has said,

"When men work, they work.
When men pray, God works."

We must love the people we minister to enough to pray for them, *and/or* pray for them until we love them enough to sacrificially minister to them. It is a good idea to get together with like-hearted Christian workers to bring before the Lord our specific questions and concerns for the individuals and the overall ministry. Remember to be sensitive to confidential concerns while praying in a group. The Scripture is filled with effective prayers that are still heard by our Lord (**Ephesians 3:16-19, Colossians 1:9, Philippians 1:9**). He knows all things and has promised to give all we ask for, when we are doing His will **(John 15:8)**.

> May our Heavenly Father's kingdom come and His perfect will be done, in every nursing home, for His glory and honor, Amen!

When I first started to work in Long Term Care, I saw firsthand how powerful spiritual care could be for the residents. One of my residents, Mary B., was very old, dependent, and non-responsive to others. We would sit her up in a wheelchair each day, but she kept her eyes closed and didn't speak. When the care team from a little evangelistic church would come every Sunday afternoon, Mary B. would get wheeled in to sit through their service. Afterwards, the volunteers would wheel her back and we would put her back to bed for a nap. After several weeks of "attendance" at the service, Mary B. was put back to bed as usual. Soon afterward, I heard a noise coming from her room. As I got closer, I could hear this resident singing to herself: "Jesus loves me, this I know..." This non-responsive resident had responded to the love of Jesus!
Pat Schlegelmilch

THE SPIRITUAL NEEDS OF NURSING-HOME RESIDENTS

The primary purpose of nursing home ministry is to help meet the spiritual needs of the residents. It is therefore of utmost importance for nursing-home missionaries to have a basic understanding of what the residents' spiritual needs are and how we can help met them. Everyone has spiritual needs. Spiritual needs cannot be met by a plush environment, a nutritionally balanced meal, a consistent exercise program or higher education. Although all these things may have a positive impact on one's life, they cannot nurture or sustain our spirit.

Fully meeting the spiritual needs of people is something only the Lord can do in the life of those who desire it. He does, however, use **us,** His ambassadors, in the process. As we help unbelievers turn to Jesus, and also help believers to abide in Christ, **He** will satisfy their spiritual hunger. Sometimes they tell us things that help us to realize that our ministry is having a positive impact in their lives.

Quotes from residents:

"My family wants me to move to Florida, but I don't want to leave . . . I have so many friends here."

"You will never know how much your visits mean to me."

"I didn't want to get up for the Bible study tonight, but now I'm so glad I did."

"You give the best medicine."

"I don't know what I would do without you."

"Before I came to this place, I was planning to end my life, but coming here was the best thing that ever happened to me. I found God in this place."

"I love to come to your church services. You make things so clear and understandable."

"I used to be afraid to die, but now I'm ready."

Following is a brief summary of the five primary spiritual needs you will encounter in your outreach: friendships, faith, hope, peace and purpose. There are certainly other spiritual needs that people have, but we believe you will discover that as these five core needs are met, your friends will also find fulfillment in most other areas as well.

1. Caring Friendships

Caring friendships are about having someone who cares and someone to care for. This is brotherly love. Most nursing home residents have outlived their spouses and friends. Their families may be out of town or worse yet, unwilling to visit. An estimated 80% of nursing home residents do not receive regular visits from family or past friends. This is sometimes due to unresolved conflicts that have damaged their relationships. Regardless of the reasons, nursing home residents are lonely and are very hungry for the personal attention friendships can provide.

Caring friendships tie in with all spiritual needs. It is the platform for <u>all</u> successful ministry. Caring friendships provide the compassion, encouragement and support needed to sustain a person.

> *Personal relationships with the residents are what transform a ministry-care team from **doing** a ministry to **being** a ministry.*

We all have gifts to give **(1 Corinthians 12:4-11)**. The gifts of time, encouragement and kind words are so valuable and must never be underestimated. Friendships find their beginning when someone gives their gift to one who will receive it.

Another gift we can constantly share in the care center (in fact wherever we go), is the Word of God. Our caring friendship will be the first message of God's love that a resident will hear. When this *initial* message of God's love is loud and clear, our friends will also desire to hear the rest of the message found in His written Word. As our gifts are respectfully offered, they become the receiver's greatest treasures.

And now I will show you the most excellent way. If I speak in the tongues of men and of angels, but have not love, I am only a resounding gong or a clanging cymbal. If I have the gift of prophecy and can fathom all mysteries and all knowledge, and if I have a faith that can move mountains, but have not love, I am nothing (1 Corinthians 12:31-13:2).

I (Bill) have an 89-year-old friend whom for the past eight years I have visited several times a month. About two years ago, she had a mild stroke that has caused her to become disoriented and very mentally frail. While sitting with her the other day, I asked, "What is the most important thing that you can tell me about your life?" I really did not think she would give me much of an answer. But she was right on when she slowly replied, "Right now ----- to be liked".

Scriptures on caring friendships: **1 Samuel 18:1 & 20:17, Ruth 1:16, Proverbs 17:17, Ecclesiastes 4:9-11, Matthew 22:39, John 13:1-17, 13:34-35 & 15:13, Colossians 3:12-14, Hebrews 13:2, 1 John 4:7-21.**

2. Faith in God

For God so loved the world that He gave His only begotten Son, that whosoever believes in Him would not perish but have everlasting life (John 3:16).

Faith is accepting, as fact, the things we cannot see or feel. When people lack faith in God (The Father, Jesus and the Holy Spirit), they have no foundation for any spiritual fulfillment. Faith in Jesus enables people to embrace His grace and righteousness and enter into a personal and everlasting relationship with God. Faith is not only for salvation, it is the beginning of all spiritual fulfillment.

Our friends in nursing homes need a faith in Jesus that goes beyond acknowledging that He exists. They need a faith that trusts that Jesus will do what He has promised, a faith that will trust Him enough to pray and do what He says to do. They need to be encouraged to take steps of faith that will help them grow closer to God by letting go of the things that hinder their relationship with Him.

Faith comes from hearing the Word of the Lord Jesus **(Romans 10:17)**. Our friends need to hear that Word on a "down-to-earth" level, but not without deep respect and purity. They also need to be challenged and encouraged to practically apply the Word, even though they may feel weak spiritually or have physical limitations. Faith also comes from experiencing God's personal intervention. As our friends hear testimonies of God's faithfulness from the Word, from other residents and from us, they will be encouraged to take steps of faith.

We live by faith, not by sight (2 Corinthians 5:7).

Scriptures on faith in God: **Proverbs 3:5-6Matthew 17:20, Mark 9:23, Luke 17:5 & 18:27, John 6:28-29, 2 Corinthians 4:18, Ephesians 2:8, Hebrews 11:1-40, James 1:6-7, 1Peter 1:6-7, 1 John 5:4**

3. Enduring Hope

Hope is an eager expectation of good. When a person believes that there is nothing good in store for him, he lacks hope. People cannot live without hope. Hope enables us to confidently look beyond the present challenges, anticipating better days or better situations ahead **(Romans 8:18)**. It enables a person to wait, to persevere, and to accept difficulties and changes with an acknowledgement of God's sovereignty and providence. Hope is an anchor for the soul in the midst of a stormy sea **(Hebrews 6:18-19)**.

Unfortunately, many people have put their hope in things that God **has not** promised. When their hopes and dreams are not fulfilled, their hearts may despair and become deeply troubled **(Proverbs 13:12)**. We can encourage our friends to put their hope in the Lord Jesus and the things He **has** promised. This is done by intently listening to them and then sharing God's promises in relation to their situations and concerns. As they embrace the fact that Jesus personally loves them, and that He is faithful in keeping His covenant with those who put their trust in Him; they will gain a living hope **(1 Peter 1:3)**.

> *I pray also that the eyes of your heart may be enlightened in order that you may know the hope to which he has called you, the riches of his glorious inheritance in the saints, and his incomparably great power for us who believe (Ephesians 1:18-19a).*

Scriptures on hope: **Psalm 42:11 & 119:114, Isaiah 40:28-31, Romans 4:18, 5:4, 8:24-25, 15:4 & 13, 1 Corinthians 13:13, Colossians 1:27, 1 Timothy 5:5 & 6:17, Hebrews 7:19 & 10:23**

4. Internal Peace

Peace is rest for the soul. When a person believes he must maintain complete control over his life and/or others lives, he will lack peace. Peace allows us to rest in quiet confidence regardless of our surroundings. God's peace will guard the hearts and minds of those who put their complete trust in Christ Jesus **(Philippians 4:4-9)**.

Many people seek to gain peace by making external adjustments to their surroundings. Although adjustments should be made when appropriate, these do not usually provide internal peace. When a person seeks peace only through external methods, he forfeits the contentment the Lord really wants for him.

By praying and sharing Scriptures related to their issues and concerns, we can help our friends realize the areas in life we are responsible to control, versus the areas only the Lord is responsible to control. Encouraging them to look to Jesus, to completely trust in Him and to obey His Word, will help them enter into the perfect peace He promised to give His children **(Isaiah 26:3)**.

> *Jesus said, "Come to me, all you who are weary and burdened, and I will give you rest. Take my yoke upon you and learn from me, for I am gentle and humble in heart, and you will find rest for*

your souls. For my yoke is easy and my burden is light" (Matthew 11:28-30).

> God grant me the serenity to accept the things I cannot change; the courage to change the things I can; and the wisdom to know the difference.

Scriptures on peace: **Psalm 4:8, Isaiah 48:22 & 54:10, Jeremiah 6:16, John 14:27 & 16:33, Romans 5:1, 14:19, 15:13 & 10:17, Ephesians 2:14-17 & 4:3, Colossians 3:15, James 3:18**

5. Genuine Purpose

Purpose gives people a reason to live. When a person believes he is not needed, or that he has no value, he will lack purpose. Purpose gives us significance and value.

Nursing-home residents are people who had previously made significant contributions in their lifetime: as parents, employees, neighbors, church leaders, etc. Now they are in an environment where almost everything, including meals, laundry and daily events, are all managed by others. Unless they can become active in caring for others, they are missing a vital link in their relationship with God.

Once a person has received Christ as Savior, God commands him to live a life of love, and apart from this our faith is dead **(James 2:14-26)**. It may seem as if there is nothing many residents can do, however, we can encourage them to look beyond their own needs and interests and consider the needs of others around them **(Philippians 2:4-8)**.

We can encourage our nursing home friends to begin daily to do at least one good thing for someone else. Introducing them to other residents can help initiate relationships that might present legitimate needs; prayer, kind words, hugs and inviting others to church, are all ways they can care for others. As they reach out in love, their faith will grow and they will find genuine purpose and experience the joy of the Lord **(John 15:10-13)**.

A note of caution: It is very important to be sensitive to the resident's physical and mental conditions. What may seem to be a small task to us could be a major task for a frail senior. Also, people sometimes hesitate reaching out to others because they fear rejection. Be patient, expect delays and keep pouring on encouragement.

For we are God's workmanship, created in Christ Jesus to do good works, which God prepared in

> *It is when the residents begin to genuinely care for each other that the nursing home is transformed from an institution for the terminally ill to a life-giving community.*

advance for us to do (Ephesians 2:10).

Scriptures on purpose: **Micah 6:8, Psalm 92:12, Matthew 5:16, Acts 17:26, 1 Corinthians 12:21-26, 2 Corinthians 9:6-13, Titus 3:14, Hebrews 6:10, 1 Peter 2:12, James 2:14-26, Philemon 1:6**

Joining the Lord in meeting these spiritual needs is the primary purpose for nursing-home ministry. We therefore want to encourage you to study these spiritual needs and the Scriptures provided to learn how you can specifically help your friends live a more fulfilled life.

We recommend that missionaries who are new to this field first develop discernment and skills in establishing caring friendships, and then set realistic goals for expanding into the other four. Remember: if all you ever do in a care center is go room-to-room to spend five or ten minutes with a few residents, you would be doing a great work! This overview of spiritual needs is shared to allow nursing-home missionaries to develop their ministry beyond casual visits. We are hopeful that the beginner will not be overwhelmed. Just be there for the people and grow at your own pace. As you abide in Christ, and point seekers to Him, He will meet their spiritual needs.

If you remain in me and my words remain in you, ask whatever you wish, and it will be given you. This is to my Father's glory, that you bear much fruit, showing yourselves to be my disciples (John 15:7-8).

EVANGELISM IN THE NURSING HOME

Carl had a reputation for slugging nursing assistants and yelling up a storm. I do not think he had any friends in the nursing home. He was dreaded by most of the nurses and assistants. We (Bill and Mary Ann) were cautious not to get too close, but often greeted him with respect. One evening Carl accepted our invitation to attend our Tuesday evening Bible study. He could not talk very well but if he did not want to do something, he could make his dissatisfaction perfectly clear. When I (Bill) asked permission to take him to the Bible study, the staff at the nurse's station opened their eyes wide and said, "Oh, yes, take him!" I think they were amazed that I asked, and figured I would be bringing him back once he realized where I was taking him.

There were times during the singing that he would make a lot of noise but during the message he was fairly quiet. After several Bible studies, Carl's heart seemed to soften toward my wife and me, but I knew that he was still being aggressive with the staff.

One day on my way to visit in the home, I asked the Lord to lead me to those He wanted me to visit that day. After several routine visits with some friends, I somehow found myself kneeling next to Carl (within slugging distance). In my heart, I felt it was time to ask him about his relationship with the Lord. I could not understand all that he said, but I could make out that he was receiving my company and words. When I asked him if he wanted to pray, he nodded and followed my lead with a mumbled prayer.

Having Carl pray with me that day was a great experience, because as I first knelt next to him, I did not know if I was kneeling for him to receive salvation or for me to receive a black eye. I am certain that our relationship had made the difference.

The following week one of the nursing assistants said to me, "I don't know what you did to Carl last week but he was trying to sing Christmas carols all afternoon." I think he did not remember any of the hymns but he did not let that stop him from singing praise for his joy that the Lord had come. Carl did not completely turn from his aggression but he made a significant improvement and continued to sing at our Bible studies. A few months later, Carl went to his eternal home. I look forward to greeting him (without fear of harm) when I also arrive Home.

"Evangelism in the Nursing Home" is a topic about which there has been considerable discussion and it is an important one. There are many who believe that our main purpose in visitation should be to befriend the elderly and help meet their physical and emotional needs, offering spiritual guidance only if it is requested. Others stress the priority of direct evangelism and desire to submit all other aims to this one overarching purpose. Elderly people are so near to death, this latter group claims, that we must constantly proclaim verbally the gospel and urge repentance, lest they perish eternally.

Coming to terms with these two different points of view is no easy task. Granted, many people you visit are facing imminent death. This does not mean, however, that there is not *enough* time for the Holy Spirit to work. Overzealous evangelists who proclaim the gospel without first becoming acquainted with the person and accurately determining true needs can often do more harm than good. The good news of Jesus Christ is a gift and it must be offered as a gift, not used as a threat or a weapon.

On the other hand, sickness, an imminent operation, loneliness, grief or depression can all bring forth or make people aware of their own deep spiritual needs that can be met by the gospel as it is offered, even by someone formerly unknown to the sufferer. We must be sensitive to the fact that God has perhaps prepared someone for us to share the gospel with, and we must be ready to give the gift that has been so freely given to us.

There is no single answer as to when and how to evangelize. The key to discovering what to do in any given situation is in discerning the leading of the Holy Spirit. God has gone before us and we must respond to what He has already done and is continuing to do in people's hearts.

Our response at times may be simply showing God's love through our actions. We may also have the opportunity to share the gospel verbally. In either case, we must be people of prayer who are actively relying on God's guidance before, during, and after our visits.

As we seek to be guided in our ministry, we must not overlook the fact that God has given each of us different gifts. Some people are skilled in developing friendships and can make a lasting impression of God's love and care simply through a long, committed friendship. Others have gifts for sharing the gospel directly with people whom they don't know. Evaluate God's gifts to you, making sure you are truly honest in your motivation. On the one hand, the "friend" must not hold back from sharing the good news of Christ for fear of being thought foolish. The "evangelist," on the other hand, should not avoid making friends for fear of becoming involved and committed. With these thoughts in mind, consider the following suggestions:

- A worship service for believers can be an evangelistic service for the unconverted. The simple, direct gospel shared throughout a service is an encouragement and comfort for believers and a call to faith for non-believers. A good sermon should help the Christians in the service grow but could also include a clear review of the gospel message, followed by an invitation for anyone who is not a believer to accept Christ.
- In individual visitation, in the context of an established, caring relationship, one good way to open conversation is to share some recent insight or activity of God in your life.

    I (Bill) do not always know when it is the right time to encourage my friend to repent and invite Jesus into his heart. Of course, there is no pat answer for this, except that only the Lord knows for sure, so I try to discern what the Holy Spirit is saying to my heart. When I think it is time, I sometimes share my thirty-second testimony: "Several years ago I found myself in a terrible mess. My whole life was so messed up that I did not want to live. A friend of mine encouraged me to pray a special prayer to ask Jesus to come into my heart and be my Lord and my Savior. It was one of the greatest prayers I ever prayed and was the beginning of a growing relationship with God." Then I ask, "Have you ever prayed a prayer like that?" Their response tells me if it is time.

- Literature provides another avenue for evangelism. It is most effective when personally shared before leaving it. Avoid, when possible, mass distribution of literature without personal contact.
- Be sensitive to the needs of the individual you are visiting. These needs, which may often be very near the

surface, can provide a wonderful opportunity to express the truth and compassion of Jesus Christ.

- Sharing openly with a Christian resident in a room where there are non-Christians present can be another effective method of evangelism. We have found great interest among roommates when they see the joy and peace that a relationship with God, through Christ, can bring. Sometimes there may be only a desire to be noticed, but that, too, offers a chance to befriend and share more openly. Encourage Christian residents to share their faith with other residents who do not know Christ.

- Although our methods for evangelism with the elderly are unique in some respects, the core principles for evangelism are the same with any other person. Therefore, we recommend the reading and study of any good book on the topic.

Remember that all spiritual needs are fundamentally fulfilled only through Christ Jesus. Our role is merely to encourage people to accept Jesus' offer to come to Him and take His hand so that He can lead them along the narrow path, which leads to fulfillment of all the Father's good purposes.

Jesus works in and through us as a Christian friend. Our desire to help the residents will usually compel us to dig deeper into God's Word and to seek more diligently the Kingdom of God and His righteousness. As we press in, our Lord will freely impart more and more of His eternal treasures to share. Our presence, including our words and deeds, become the vehicle God uses to share His heavenly treasures. These treasures are hidden from the world, but because we are God's children, we share in them. What a privilege!

> *At that time Jesus, full of joy through the Holy Spirit, said, "I praise you, Father, Lord of heaven and earth, because you have hidden these things from the wise and learned, and revealed them to little children. Yes, Father, for this was your good pleasure (Luke 10:21).*

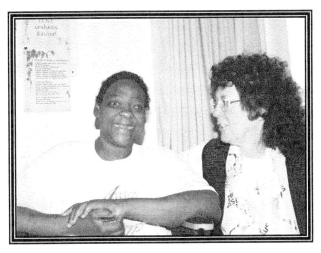

Jesus said, "By this all men will know that you are my disciples, if you love one another" (John 13:35).

CHAPTER 4

ONE-TO-ONE VISITING

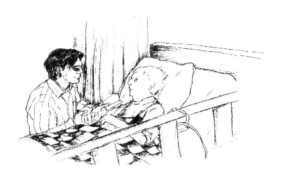

"Your visits mean more to me than I can say. Before I entered this place I was somebody, but now I am something. It took all my life to become the somebody I was, but now ill health and this institution takes who I was away and makes me just another resident. However, I want you to know that when you visit me, I become someone. I can tell that I am someone because of the way you treat me and that you're not in a hurry to end your visit with me. Thank you, I love you, too."

A nursing home resident

~~~ * ~~~

I left my nursing home friend for an extended vacation. While I was gone, I replaced my weekly visits with postcards.

"Did you get my postcards?" I asked on my return. "Oh yes!" she replied with a grin, and recited everything I had written on those cards. She has traveled with me vicariously and treasured those weekly assurances that I hadn't forgotten her.

<div align="right">Ruth Swartz</div>

In nursing homes, there is a great need to share with the residents on an individual basis. Church services and Bible studies are a very important part of nursing-home ministry; however, less than fifty percent of nursing-home residents participate in such activities. Even those who participate in the group ministry need personal fellowship. Because of the need for both types of ministry, some care teams alternate every other week between one-to-one visits and a group ministry. In this chapter, you will find numerous practical suggestions concerning visitation.

WHAT IS VISITATION?

When we consider visiting someone, we tend to think of dropping in to say hello, catching up on the latest news or just finding out how someone is. Our ideas of visiting may often boil down to making a brief appearance or exchanging a few words. The concept of visitation in the Bible is much richer.

The concept of "visit" is found in **Psalm 8:4**, where the wonder of a mighty God caring for insignificant human beings is discussed. God is mindful of us; God cares for and visits us. When Jesus came into the world, He tarried until His mission—or visit! —fulfilled the Father's will. In **Matthew 25:36,** visiting seems to imply caring for the needs of someone who is unable to care for himself. This idea is further elaborated in **James 1:27**, where doing what God commands is seen in terms of caring for orphans and widows in their distress. Visitation implies a deep devotion, evidenced by a practical demonstration of Christ's love.

Love for Christ should be our supreme motivation for visiting the elderly. Our concern and our desire to care for and protect others depends on our love for the Christ who loves us **(I John 4:20)**. As we learn more about visiting the elderly, we are really learning more about loving God **(Matthew 25:36, 40)**.

GUIDELINES FOR VISITATION

Pleasant manners and a good understanding should characterize our visits in nursing homes. As servants of our Lord Jesus, we must be willing to make necessary adjustments for the sake of honoring and helping our older friends. A good motto for nursing-home ministry could be:

"Whatever is best for the residents and honoring to the Lord.".

Embracing a motto such as this will help us to be teachable, flexible and ultimately very fruitful. Here, we list several "Be" guidelines to provide a good structure for an effective visitation ministry.

WHAT TO BE:

Be Healthy: It is a good idea to visit the nursing home well rested. Do not visit a nursing home if you have a cold, fever or other contagious illness. A minor case of sniffles to you can become life-threatening pneumonia to a nursing-home resident.

Be Neat and Clean: Pleasant-colored casual clothing is recommended. Extreme fashions can be distracting and perfumes can sometimes be irritating for people with allergies or sensitive noses. It is better to err on the formal side. Children and youth will probably need clear guidance about a "nursing-home dress code."

Be Respectful: Be sure to knock before you enter the room. Remember, the room of a nursing-home resident is now his home. Ask permission to sit. Avoid sitting on his bed. Call the resident by his name. Titles like "Honey" and "Sweetie" may spring from a kind heart but are sometimes taken as insults. We recommend that you ask them their name, and use the name they give you. Otherwise, or if you are unsure, use Mr., Mrs., or Miss. Also, try your best to get on eye level with your friend. This is less threatening and will aid in holding a conversation.

Be Aware: Each resident is a person, created in the image of God. Each resident is unique, formed by traditions and cultures that may be different from your own. Regardless of their physical, emotional or spiritual condition, they each have a personality with hurts, concerns and hidden treasures of wisdom and knowledge that they long to share.

Be Knowledgeable: All residents have rights guaranteed to them under federal and state/provincial laws, for example, the rights to privacy and confidentiality. Residents' rights are posted in every nursing home. In addition, each home has specific policies and procedures that help to govern the facility. It is important for you to understand the ones that apply to you. Learn what you can from reading other books and sharing with people who have experience in this ministry.

Be Safe: Years ago, it was acceptable for a volunteer to feed a resident or help transfer them from a bed to a chair or from one chair to another. Over the past years however, new laws have gone into effect that generally prohibit visitors from assisting with these activities. What sometimes may seem to be a helping hand to residents and staff may be a violation of state/federal laws. These laws protect residents from harm, like choking or a fall; they also protect you, as a visitor, from liability. Check with the home(s) you visit if you have questions, as rules may vary slightly from place to place.

There is also a need to wash your hands frequently and thoroughly to prevent the spread of germs, especially during cold and flu season. Towelettes and waterless hand-washes are great items to carry with you for preventing the spread of infectious germs.

Be a Good Listener: Good listening skills go a long way in the nursing home. Sometimes we think we must carry the conversation; however, the more we can sit back and attentively listen, the more our friend is likely to sense that we care. We must also listen to the Holy Spirit who can direct our conversation with wit and wisdom as well as guide us to a consideration of spiritual and eternal things.

Be Patient: Be focused on the friend you are visiting and not in a hurry to meet long-term goals or to move on to the next visit. Though your desire may be to share the Word and pray with a resident, it may take several visits and a developing friendship before a resident is open to this. A skillful fisherman knows how to wait and try different approaches to reach his goals. There may also be people you visit who will never want you to read Scripture or pray with them. Respect their right to this.

Be Helpful: Be willing to help in whatever practical ways are appropriate, such as reading or writing a letter, cleaning eyeglasses or adjusting a blanket. Be very careful, however, to not make changes that might counteract what the staff is doing. When in doubt, ask permission.

> *Be joyful in hope, patient in affliction, faithful in prayer.*
> **Romans 12:12**

Be Honest: If you don't know the answer to something, just say so. Sometimes a resident will say something that you cannot hear or understand. It is perfectly acceptable to say, "I'm sorry I did not hear (or understand) what you said. Could you please repeat it?" If you find it impossible to understand words, try to find alternative ways to communicate, for example through body language, voice inflection, writing, or hand squeezing. To help clarify communication, it may be helpful to say, "Did you say… ? "' or " I think you said…'". or "Did I hear you correctly?"

Be Trustworthy: If you say you are going to do something, keep your word. It is good practice to write your promises down so you do not forget them. Be careful not to make a promise you cannot keep. If asked to do something that is in violation of the home's policies, you can say, "I'm sorry, I am not allowed to do that, but I would be happy to help you turn your call light on or inform the staff of your need."

If you respectfully inform staff of a resident's needs, your input will be received much better than if you simply tell staff what to do. When approaching staff, it is better to say, "Mrs. Jones has requested help in... I told her that I would inform you". Rather than, Mrs. Jones needs..."

Be Obedient: There may be times that you mistakenly violate one of the home's policies or rules. If this should happen, apologize to the appropriate person(s). If there is a disagreement with the staff, this should be taken to your team leader and, if necessary, to whoever oversees your visits, e.g. the Activities Director or Coordinator of Volunteers. Seek clarification, but be very cautious about arguing with nursing-home staff, as such activity almost always produces negative fruit and will limit your overall effectiveness and freedom in the home. Remember that you are also a representative of your local church and of Christ our King.

Be Cheerful: Residents normally enjoy humor. Clean, happy, fun jokes can often brighten a day. Some residents may even enjoy a little teasing, but use caution and good discernment. Reckless words can hurt.

Be Able to Handle Rejection: Sometimes, a resident will not accept you. There can be many reasons for rejection that have nothing to do with you. Much of the time rejection is the result of a hard and hurting heart expressing itself. Some residents may also have had a negative experience in relation to a church in the past and may associate you with that experience. Don't take rejection personally. Through time, prayer, deeds of kindness and perseverance, hard hearts may soften. Handle rejection with grace and do not be discouraged. It will not happen very often.

Be Adaptable: Every visit will be unique in its own way. It is a good idea to have proven techniques to begin conversations and establish relationships. Keep in mind that one approach does not work for all people.

Be Faithful: The following story was taken from God Cares News November/December 1999:

> *At one of our training seminars in Kansas, an Activities Director gave a brief message that challenged us. What would it be like, she shared, if you got up Sunday morning, dressed and prepared, then drove to church, sat in your usual spot, waited for the minister to start the service, and waited, and waited, and waited, and the minister never showed up? What would you think? How might you feel? There was a man named Winston Churchill who gave a very famous speech. It is only ten words long but it was and is a very inspiring message. Churchill said; "Never give up! Never give up! Never! Never! Never! Never!" She continued, explaining that she too had a message that was only ten words long. This is a message that every activities director would agree with, because those who visit care centers to share the love and word of God are very important to the residents. The message was; "Always show up! Always show up! Always! Always! Always! Always!"*

Be Yourself: It is easy to look at all the above suggestions and feel overwhelmed or insufficient for the job. Remember, they are guidelines. Be yourself and always treat others the way you would want to be treated **(Matthew 7:12)**.

GUIDELINES FOR THE FIRST FEW VISITS

Since the first few visits are often the most challenging, it is good to be as spiritually and mentally prepared as possible. The following are some suggestions to assist you in visit preparation and goal setting. After reading and meditating on this section, feel free to branch out on your own, trusting God to prepare you, guide you and give you the flexibility you will need for each situation you encounter.

Pre-Visit Preparation

Before you go to the nursing home for the first time, and in successive visits as well, ask yourself the following questions:

1. Have I taken time to pray? Have I prayed
   - for myself and for what I will do and say
   - for those I am about to meet
   - for the staff of the home
   - for others going with me

2. Do I have a goal for today? Can I
   - help write a letter
   - talk about the Lord
   - chat with three people
   - lead a worship service

3. Do I have the material I need? These could include
   - Bible, tracts
   - large-print hymnals, devotional guides
   - games, puzzles
   - small gift(s)
   - writing materials
   - musical instrument
   -

4. How do I look? How do I feel? How do I smell?

> Is my dress appropriate and not too casual?
> Would someone want to talk to me? Do I look cheerful?
> What are my motives for visiting? Am I trying to serve God and the elderly?
> I'll be getting up close and personal to talk to people. Do I have my breath mints?

The First Visit

As mentioned earlier in this chapter, your first visits may be closely observed by the staff who are watching for genuine care and respect. In time, they will see the fruit of your labor and respond accordingly.

- Contact the nurse in charge of the unit you are visiting. It is wise to have your presence officially recognized, although that may not always be necessary. There may also be a check-in point at the front desk or in the activities office. Find out the rules and abide by them. Although checking in may seem unnecessary after a while, contact with those in charge not only is a courtesy to them, but also provides an opportunity for you to find out who is sick, depressed, lonely, and in special need of a visitor.

- When arriving at the door of an individual's room, be sure to knock and await permission to enter; or enter slowly and tentatively, especially if the person is hard of hearing. This is probably the only private space this person has, so don't violate his control over it.

- You may wish to begin visitation by meeting the person in an open lounge. This setting is good for general conversation, but often presents too many distractions for deeper, more personal talk.

- Introduce yourself and start a light, friendly conversation. Tell the person a little about yourself. Include your name, your relationship to the home, and share any possible background you might have in common, such as job or church. If you have no such common background with the individual, just state your purpose in visiting. Be honest, concerned, and direct.

- The environment in which the resident lives is very important to him and can be helpful to you for beginning a conversation. The resident's room, other people in the room, music playing in the room, a television or radio program, flowers, cards or pictures on the wall, religious items like a Bible or rosary – any of these can open up areas for conversation, as well as give clues to the internal mental and spiritual condition of the person you are visiting. Be prepared to adapt your goals to the person's needs.

- Though you do have a decidedly spiritual interest in your friends, beware of focusing too much, or even exclusively, perhaps, on "religious" things. Be ready to be involved in the totality of a person's life.

- Leave any literature that may be helpful in a particular situation. This may not always be appropriate, for example, with those who can no longer understand the written word anymore or read English. Remember that your words and actions leave the lasting impression. As you get to know residents, you will be better equipped to bring in appropriate literature, including devotionals, magazines and even books.

- If possible, tell the people you visit when they may expect to see you again. Don't promise more than you can realistically do. If you have promised to visit on a certain day and are unable to make it at the specified time, be sure to call the home and leave a message or ask to speak to the person directly on the phone.

- After you leave, write reminder notes for yourself, reflect on your visit and pray. As you await your next visit, make a note of any Scripture that may apply to the person's situation and meditate on it, praying for wisdom as to how and when to use it in subsequent visits to help meet specific needs. Ask others on the ministry team to pray for you and your "new friend." This is a great way to involve others in the ministry to the elderly; be aware, however, about issues of confidentiality. Make some tentative plans for your next and following visits, including the possibility of relating to the individual's family or involvement in other activities.

WHAT TO SAY WHEN YOU DON'T KNOW WHAT TO SAY

For many people, one of the greatest fears about visiting a nursing home revolves around the question: "What will I talk about?" With most of the people you visit this won't be a problem. The resident will do much of the talking, and you will find yourself listening to many stories from the past. But your visit with more quiet residents may require more effort. Many elderly people sit for hours or even for days on end, scarcely speaking a word or being spoken to. For them, there is little to stimulate their minds. It may be up to you to carry the conversation.

When visiting for the first time, your introduction could be: "Hi or Hello. My name is ___. I am here to visit some friends today and thought you might enjoy a friendly visit." Commenting on pictures and personal articles displayed in their rooms is a great conversation starter. Another effective tip is to always reveal something about yourself before you ask a resident a more personal question. For example: "Hi my name is ___. What is your name?"; "I'm from ___; are you originally from this area?"

We have found that people who find it difficult to lead a conversation need not fear the challenge. Most nursing-home residents are happy just to have someone visit and talk to them. What seems to matter most is that someone cares enough to spend time with them.

As mentioned earlier, one other possible concern is being asked a question to which you do not know the answer. The honest answer, "I'm sorry, I don't know," is very acceptable and usually well respected.

Helpful questions for starting conversations

Below is a list of further conversation starters. They are adapted from a newsletter, "Aging With Grace" (April 1992) by John Koppenaal. Don't feel bound to any specific method or style; feel free to use them as guidelines.

- Birthplace - Where were you born?
- Parents - Mother. - What was your mother like? Was she a good cook? What was one of her best dishes? Did she have any hobbies?
- Parents – Father - What kind of work did your father do? What did he like to do best? Did he have any hobbies?
- Children - How many children did you have? Do any of them live near by? (Note: this can be a sensitive topic for some people if they have children who do not visit; be prepared for emotional responses if you ask this question. Also, some elderly people may have outlived all of their children)
- Family - Do you have any brothers and sisters? Where do they live?
- Grandparents - What can you remember about your grandparents? Where were they born?
- Religion - What was the role of religion in your family? What church did you attend? Did you go to Sunday School? What was your favorite Bible verse or story?
- Neighborhood - What do you remember about the place where you grew up?
- School - What do you remember about your school--your favorite teacher, and the subjects you liked best?

- Growing up - How did you spend your summers? Did you have any hobbies, favorite songs, or sports?
- Work - What kind of work did you do? What did you buy with your first check?
- Entertainment - What did you do for fun growing up? What were your favorite radio programs and movies?
- Memories - What do you remember about: World War II, the Twenties, Prohibition, the Depression, Korean War, Vietnam, the Kennedy assassination, the first man on the moon?
- Politics - Who was your favorite president, and why? Who are some of the people you admire most? Why?
- Life - What have been some of the most significant changes/achievements in your lifetime? What was the happiest time of your life?

> *"People tend to lose their individuality in an institution, so it gives their egos a boost when you find something attractive about them or their 'homes.' Don't patronize; be genuine. Love them and they will love in return."*
>
> Dorothy Miller, A Song for Grandmother

We must be careful that general conversation is not so much fun for us that we neglect opportunities to bring Christ's comfort, such as by reading Scripture and/or praying with a resident. On the other hand, having a genuine interest in people is vital to establishing a caring friendship that can lead to a discussion of spiritual things. Below are some questions and comments that can open up conversation about the Lord. Keep in mind that it may take several visits before a person is open to this kind of conversation.

- Are you a member of a church? What church? What did your church/religion mean to you?
- Has your pastor been in to visit you? If no, ask: Have you notified him? Would you like me to notify him?
- Were you active in your church? What did you do?
- How does the Lord help you during time of stress or difficulty?
- Do you have any favorite Bible verses/hymns?
- What values are most important to you and that you desire to pass on to others?
- Do you feel confident that you will be with Jesus when you die? If the person says no but they would like to feel confident or, if in your conversation you sense they might be open to becoming a Christian, you might include more of your own personal testimony. For example: Several years ago, I prayed a special prayer and asked Jesus to come into my heart, to be my personal Lord and Savior. It was one of the greatest prayers I ever prayed and was the beginning of a growing relation with Him. Have you ever prayed a prayer like that? (Yes; What happened?) (No; Would you like to?)

Be careful that your questions and comments do not lead your friend to think he is being surveyed. Remember: pray, be yourself, and let your conversation flow naturally.

The Second Visit

Be sure you have reviewed your notes from the first visit. Pray and meditate on the response you think would be appropriate for the visit. Follow the same basic procedure as you did in the first visit, noting especially the following:

- Be ready for any changes that may have occurred, such as a new roommate, the death of a friend or relative, good or bad news, change of mood, and so on. Adapt the response you *thought* would be right to fit the new situation. Don't hold to a rigid agenda; be flexible.

- Enter again with an introduction that does not necessarily assume the person remembers who you are or even your prior visit. You may need to reintroduce yourself and your reason for being there. Give gracious clues to your identity as needed. Stimulating people to remember provides good mental exercise and helps establish a proper sequence and time-consciousness. Don't push too hard for recall, however, as some may have memory deficit.

- If necessary, try to undo any misunderstanding that may have arisen from the first visit. Plan not to repeat your early mistakes. Did you monopolize the conversation? Be prepared to listen more. Did you come across too forcefully in sharing the gospel? Be more sensitive this time. Were you too informal with someone with a more formal background? Be more adaptable and apologize if it's appropriate.

The Third and Following Visits

As you spend more time with an individual, you may not feel the need to take notes. If you're spending a fair amount of time (twenty to thirty minutes at least) with your friend, note taking is probably not necessary. If, however, you are visiting a large number of people for short periods of time, it's probably best to keep a few notes in order to keep everyone straight in your mind. Be guided by your own needs.

The following hints are offered as suggestions. Consider these tips as you seek to be most effective in your visits.

- **Make every visit count.** Since elderly people are close (relatively speaking) to death, and some may be sick and actually very near dying, make every visit count. Be fully present for the person, giving each one your complete, loving attention.

- **Visit in twos when possible.** This is especially helpful when you are first starting out in visiting. One can be praying while the other is sharing. It is valuable initially for a less experienced visitor to go with a more experienced person.
- **Encourage spiritual examination and life review.** Meditation on one's past life, including perceived successes and failures, may help people deal with their feelings and with unresolved concerns or conflicts. Move toward a continuing program of personal, meaningful examination of self. Things in the past cannot be changed, and dwelling on negative feelings and experiences long-term is usually not helpful or healthy; but people *can* learn from mistakes and improve present attitudes and behavior. Remember your role. You are not a pastoral counselor or psychologist. Let the resident set the pace in the process of reminiscence.
- **Don't assume that residents have physical or mental disabilities by their appearances.** Approach them as if there are no disabilities, then make adjustments as the need becomes apparent.
- **Gifts:** Residents appreciate receiving small gifts. With food and glass items there are allergy and safety concerns; staff should be consulted before you purchase such items. Sometimes a birthday card with a personal note is a perfect gift, or a large print magazine, devotional guide, church bulletin or book. The following is one example of gift-giving shared by some nursing-home visitors:

    Jan is battling an illness that keeps her at home most of the time, but she and her mother Marie are spending a lot of their time blessing nursing-home residents in a very creative way. This mother and daughter team have purchased materials and sewn together adorable teddy bears for nursing home residents. Each bear has a ribbon around its neck that says, "Jesus Loves You!" And if you press the right paw, it will play you a musical tune.

After a dozen or so are made, Marie and her husband Norm get a list of residents that do not receive outside visits. They go to the nursing home and personally deliver a bear and a blessing to each person on the list.

When asked about this ministry, Jan said, "I thought that there have got to be people who do not get visits and would appreciate something warm and fuzzy to hug. I realize that it could be me in the nursing home." Her mother Marie said, "The reactions of the residents give me such an uplifting feeling that it is worth every stitch of time invested. I feel that I am much more blessed than the residents as I see them receive the bears with such gratitude."

Over the past year, these ladies have made over eighty lovable bears. I was blessed to go with Marie and Norm last month and saw how grateful the residents were to receive a warm, fuzzy friend and a reminder that Jesus loves them and has not forgotten them.

God Cares News

- **Reading:** Many residents are no longer able to read. They sometimes appreciate having the Bible read to them. Other sources of reading are devotionals and short stories from magazines such as *Our Daily Bread, Guideposts, The Upper Room,* and *Readers Digest.* Please read slowly and project your voice. When reading Scriptures to your friend, don't just read them, share them. When possible, read from the resident's Bible (after asking permission).

- **Confidentiality:** A nursing-home resident's medical condition, treatments, and medications are confidential. It is not appropriate to ask about these. The person may, however, want to talk to you about them. Be sure to listen, but never give medical advice, and consider all personal information shared confidential.

- **Touch:** When appropriate, touch your friend's hand, head, or shoulder. Let hugs be one of the gifts you often give if a person likes being touched. Any form of touching, including hand-shakes and hugs should be gentle as some residents have arthritis or osteoporosis and often have fragile skin.

- **Music:** If you have the ability to play a small instrument like a harmonica, autoharp, or guitar, this can often be a great blessing to a resident. Music has the ability to cut through the toughest situations. Another way to bless your friends with music is to take a portable tape player into their room. After a time of fellowship, leave the player going while you visit another friend. Old hymns are especially meaningful. Keep in mind, however, that you should do this only with the resident's consent.

- **Give hope.** Sometime during the visit, offer to share the word of God and pray. It is important to have the resident's permission and to ask him if he has a special portion he would like you to read. There are, of course, exceptions when it would be inappropriate to make such an offer; for example, if they expressed negative comments against Jesus or seemed to be overly agitated when you started reading. In such cases, pray silently, entrusting your friend to the Lord, and awaiting a God-given opening for sharing.

- **Encourage active faith.** When residents reach out to others, they spend less time focusing on their own problems. Help them to love and serve their neighbors and staff members in appropriate ways, if only by prayer. The result of loving others is peace and joy.

- **Involve roommates.** On many occasions, roommates are listening to **your conversations and prayers;** sometimes they want to be included.
- **Respect the privacy curtains.** Do not open them or peer behind them without permission.
- **Consider other ways to invest.** Seek ways other than religious-focused visits to be involved in the lives of residents. Consider their needs and plan constructively and creatively to meet these needs. This may mean writing letters for them, taking them to a potluck, or arranging transportation to a church service—the possibilities are endless. See Chapter 10 for more ideas.

More good points from Tom and Kaye DePinto:

1. Let your light of love shine brighter than your Biblical knowledge.
2. Do not sit on a bed when the resident is in it.
3. If a medical problem occurs, report it at once.
4. Do not untie restraints, lower bed rails or adjust geri-chairs.
5. Talk at eye level.
6. Check with staff before running an errand.

Adapted from Ministry in Action

At first, I (Bill) thought my time given to visit my nursing-home friends was a sacrifice. Indeed, at first it was. Now, 19 years later, I see my missionary service has really been an investment that shall remain an eternal blessing.

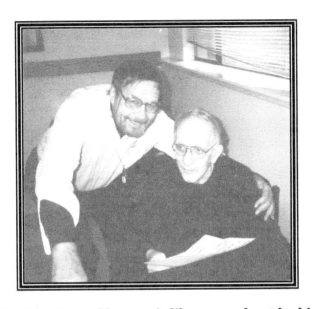

The kingdom of heaven is like a merchant looking for fine pearls. When he found one of great value, he went away and sold everything he had and bought it (Matthew 13:45-46).

CHAPTER 5

PREPARING A WAY FOR THE LORD

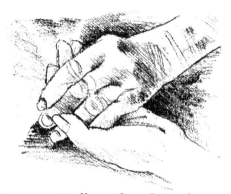

Betty cannot talk, and so I try desperately to read her lips, hanging on to each movement they make. When I asked Betty what religion she was, she wrote "Christmas" on a pad of paper. She obviously meant 'Christian.' I asked her if she knew Jesus and she assured me she did. When I first placed the headphones on her and turned on some hymns, this lady rose up and tears almost came to her eyes. She kept grabbing my hand and patting it. It's like she had an injection of a renewed life! I have found that the use of this tape player with headphones at a volume comfortable for the listener is a marvelous tool.

Carol Horn

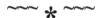

One day I visited a house where our sisters shelter the aged. This was one of the nicest houses in England, filled with beautiful and precious things, yet there was not one smile on the faces of those people. All of them were looking toward the door.

I asked the sister in charge, "Sister, why doesn't anybody smile? Why do they look constantly at the door?"

"The same thing always happens," she answered. "They are always waiting for someone to come to visit them. They dream of a son or daughter, some member of the family, or a friend coming through that door to visit them."

Loneliness was an expression of their poverty, the poverty of seeing themselves abandoned by relatives and friends.

Mother Teresa, Heart of Joy

RISING ABOVE DENOMINATIONAL WALLS

There are many denominations represented in the nursing home. When we banner the title of any particular denomination in the home, including our own, we risk limiting our sphere of influence among both the residents and staff. Although a spirit of unity is growing throughout the Christian church, some people still think it is best to avoid any contact with people from denominations other than their own. As missionaries and ambassadors of Christ in nursing homes, we do well to leave our denominational differences at our church and focus on the things we have in common. When asked what church we are from, a good reply could be, "I attend _____ Church. Do you have a church in this area?" If the person goes to a Christian church, you can look for commonalities. You can also say, "We go to different churches, but we have the same Heavenly Father".

Another challenge you will face in a nursing home is sharing with someone who believes things that you *know* to be contrary to what the Lord has taught us in Scripture. During such discussions, you may want to **respectfully** offer words of correction. If you sense that your relationship is not strong enough to warrant this, simply listen to the other person and move on to another subject, rather than argue a point. Whether the person is a believer or not, our ultimate goal is to focus on things that will encourage him to take steps of faith toward Jesus. God's promise to Christians is that the Holy Spirit will lead and guide him into all truth; this same Spirit can work in the lives of non-believers to draw them to Jesus Christ.

> *"Teacher, which is the greatest commandment in the Law?" Jesus replied: "'Love the Lord your God with all your heart and with all your soul and with all your mind.' This is the first and greatest commandment. And the second is like it: 'Love your neighbor as yourself.' All the Law and the Prophets hang on these two commandments."*
> **Matthew 22:36-40**

We can learn a great principle from the story of the apostle Paul in Athens recorded in **Acts 17:16-34**. Even though Paul was distressed by the people's idolatry, he looked for common ground to lay a foundation for truth. When given permission to speak, Paul began by saying,

> *"Men of Athens! I see that in every way you are very religious. . .I even found an altar with this inscription: To an unknown God. Now what you worship as something unknown I am going to proclaim to you."*

Notice that Paul did not focus on what was wrong with their belief system. Instead he respectfully sought to build a foundation on things he had in common with them, i.e. an interest in spiritual things and desire to worship. Paul then used his own knowledge of Scripture to reveal a true understanding of God.

As Christians (Catholic, Protestant, or Orthodox), we have much common ground for conversation. For starters, here are

fourteen things that almost every Christian believer will agree with:
- God is the Creator of the heavens and the earth.
- Jesus is the Son of God the Father.
- Jesus Christ is LORD.
- Jesus was born of the Virgin Mary.
- Jesus suffered under Pontius Pilate.
- Jesus died on the cross for the sins of the whole world.
- Jesus rose from the dead.
- Jesus ascended into heaven.
- Jesus is the way, the truth and the life – the only way to heaven.
- Jesus sits at God the Father's right hand.
- Jesus can and will embrace those who call upon His name in faith.
- Jesus gives His Holy Spirit to believers.
- Jesus commands us to repent from our sins.
- The Bible is God's Holy Word.

The words to the Apostle's Creed are also usually accepted by persons from various denominations: The traditional English version reads:

I believe in God the Father Almighty, Maker of heaven and earth. And in Jesus Christ his only Son our Lord; who was conceived by the Holy Ghost, born of the Virgin Mary, suffered under Pontius Pilate, was crucified, died and was buried; he descended into hell; the third day he rose again from the dead; he ascended into heaven, and sitteth at the right hand of God the Father Almighty; from thence he shall come to judge the quick and the dead. I believe in the Holy Ghost; the holy catholic (or Christian) Church;

the communion of saints; the forgiveness of sins; the resurrection of the body; and the life everlasting. AMEN.

When we are keeping our focus on Jesus and the fundamental truths found in Scripture, we will find much common ground on which to build relationships in Christ. We should not seek common ground, however, at the expense of compromising fundamental truths, such as those mentioned above. However, we may need to lay aside some of our traditions, beliefs or methods of worship so that others would not be hindered from seeing Jesus. A good saying to keep in mind is:

*In the Name of Jesus Christ our LORD,
let us seek unity in essentials,
liberty in non-essentials,
charity in all things.*

When people have been affiliated with one particular denomination all their lives, certain beliefs can become a part of their identity. It is important, therefore, to realize that they may not even know or understand many of the deeper theological beliefs of their own denomination. When they express strong concerns about certain doctrines or beliefs, they are not so much defending their denomination, but their own integrity, culture or identity.

Laying aside our differences does not mean that we are ashamed of our personal religious beliefs, but for the sake of charity, we never push them. The Apostle Paul wrote, ***"I have become all things to all men so that by all possible means I might save some" (1Corinthians 9:22).*** Therefore, to the Baptist, Methodist, Catholic, or Pentecostal, let us become Baptist, Methodist, Catholic, or Pentecostal, that we might help draw them into a closer relationship with Jesus, who died for us all-- that we might be One in Him.

Do not cause anyone to stumble, whether Jews, Greeks or the church of God--even as I try to

please everybody in every way. For I am not seeking my own good but the good of many, so that they may be saved. (1Corinthians 10:32-33)

LISTENING WITH YOUR HEART – RESPONDING IN LOVE

Listening is a skill that is vitally important to effective communication. This is true not only in nursing-home ministry, but also to all our relationships in life. Listening shows you really care and also accept the other person for who he is. A good listener learns about the other person's interests, hopes, needs, and desires, and gains insights for being helpful in these areas. For most of us, listening is a skill that needs to be developed.

When we listen with our hearts, we are seeking to hear not only the words a person is trying to say, but also the message behind the words. This involves paying close attention to more than the words spoken; it also involves reading body language, being sensitive to tone of voice, and interpreting the meaning of eye contact or lack thereof. Listening also involves interpreting times of silence. The person who listens values "*seeking to understand*" before "*being understood.*"

As visitors in the nursing home, we may think we must always contribute a profound instructive response to our friend's comments and concerns. However, a listening ear may be appreciated much more. In reality, most people, when they reflect on past visits, will remember the visitor's heart attitude more than any words that were shared.

Several months ago I (Bill) stopped by to visit one of my friends in the nursing home. He has been there for a few years and has never completely adjusted to these major changes.

"Jim! How are you doing?" I asked. Jim's reply was slow and gloomy; "Oooh ... old."

Just the other day Jim was sitting in his wheelchair in the hall. I was trying to hurry along for a four o-clock meeting. As I was passing by, Jim said, "Hey, can you help me?" I stopped, stooped down and greeted him. He was so sad, but when he realized who I was, he gave a smile and said. "Oh ... it's you! ... You know ... everything is not good." Then putting his hand on my arm he said, "Except you," and smiled again. After a few minutes I stood up and headed for my meeting. I thought to myself, "I almost missed the best meeting of my day!"

How do you know if you are a good listener? Ask your family, friends, or coworkers; they are usually your best and most honest critics! The fruit of good listening is that people want to be around you. They want to share with you because they sense you care.

Below are a few questions to test your listening skills. When someone is talking to me, do I:

- find myself wanting to answer before they finish their statement or question?
- lose track of what they are saying?
- tend to give a pat answer to fix their problem?
- become impatient and/or fidgety?
- take control of the conversation?
- think about other things that are more important to me?

Answering "Yes" to any of these questions is a good sign that reviewing the following six tips for being a good listener could be a blessing to you and also your nursing-home friends. There is no secret to quality listening; it just takes a few purposeful steps and practice.

1. **Choose to listen** - Have genuine concern for your friend. Quality listening is work at first but will soon become a natural part of your communication.
2. **Prayerfully listen** - Pray a silent prayer, asking the Lord to help you hear and understand what is really being said. Prayer is your greatest resource.
3. **Listen with empathy** - In empathetic listening, we are seeking to lean into our friend's emotions, thoughts, and feelings. We intently listen to feel and understand their words and emotions in depth. Our body language will also communicate that we are listening: We can get at eye level and position ourselves in the line of sight of our friend so he does not have to turn his head too much to see us. Lean towards your friend. If your friend begins to cry, you may want to take his hand to comfort him.
4. **Ask questions or respond with interest** - This helps us clarify what our friend is saying and encourages him to talk more and truly share his concerns. We can use statements or questions like:
    - "That's interesting,"
    - "What's on your mind?"
    - "Tell me more about it,"
    - "Is there anything else?" or
    - "Your thoughts are important to me."
5. **Rephrase what you think your friend is saying to clarify their heart's message** - When you rephrase a person's message you are saying, "This is what I understand you are saying." We try to do this with some of the main points that our friend makes. This will often aid him in communicating his message too. Rephrasing statements normally start with words like:
    - "It sounds like…"
    - "You feel…"
    - "Do you mean…?".

6. **Prayerfully discern an instructive response** - Ask the Lord, "What is the need here? How can I bless my friend?" At this point, treat your friend the way you would want to be treated if you were in their situation. In doing so, you can be confident that your response will most often be beneficial.

> *People don't care what you know, until they know that you care.*
>
> *People will remember the fruit of your heart more than the words of your mouth. If your fruit is love, joy, peace, patience, kindness, goodness, gentleness, and self-control, your words will be much more effective.*

Remember the following:

- Sometimes people are not looking for answers but are only hoping for a listening ear. Silence, a hug, or an expression of concern may be the best response for this visit. The next visit may be more instructive. Take your time. Don't try to fix someone's lifelong problem in 15 minutes.

- Sometimes our words have no effect, but sincere prayer always does, even though we may not see the Lord's intervention initially.

- We may need to persevere through a time of tears. In most cases, the release of deep feelings is therapeutic and may enable our friend to release their burdens.

- One of the best exercises for being an excellent listener is not to open your mouth (**James 1:19**).

- Our words can bring life or death. Timing is critical. The book of Proverbs is full of help in this area: (**Proverbs 10:19, 11:9, 11:12, 12:6, 18 & 25, 15:4, 15:30, 18:13, 18:21, 20:5, 30:6**).

- The Holy Spirit is the counselor and comforter. Let Him use you to bring life.
- Honest words like "That must really hurt you" or "You have really been through a lot" can help, but avoid saying "I know how you feel." Although you may understand your friend's concerns, and may even have had a similar situation in your life, only he and the LORD know how he feels, **(Proverbs 14:10).**

HOW DO WE LEAD A RESIDENT TO JESUS?

Jesus said; *"Come to Me...."(Matthew 11:28).* As we come, He promises to take care of us. But how can we effectively help people come or turn to Jesus? There are many "plans of salvation" that have been very effective in helping millions of people make decisions to follow Christ, but sometimes these do not work as well in a nursing-home setting because of the many different religious backgrounds and levels of cognitive impairment. There will be times when residents will be very open to the gospel. You may be able to lead them down preplanned evangelistic paths using tools like the "Roman Road," or the "Four Spiritual Laws;" on the other hand these may become confusing for them or cause you to lose their attention. The following points may prove to be very liberating not only in nursing homes, but also in the church, family, and even one's own life.

How to lead a person to Jesus:

Prayerfully: Sometimes our efforts are fruitless because they are also prayerless. By prayer, we mean making requests and listening to what God may say in response to our prayer. Through prayer, God leads us to do things at the right time and sometimes in ways we have never thought of doing.

As a friend: It is possible to lead strangers to Jesus, and some people have special gifts of evangelism and are able to do this quite easily, but in a nursing-home context, friendship evangelism is the most effective way for a person to become a Christian. Friendship earns us the right and privilege to be heard and to share the gospel. In truth, we are actually helpers to those who are seekers of Christ. Whether saved or unsaved, a seeker/helper relationship is, in reality, two or more seekers of truth sharing and helping each other along the journey to Jesus.

With understanding: We need to understand what it means to lead someone to Jesus. If Jesus had His throne nearby and we could take our struggling friend by the hand and walk him to His door, we would knock, gain access, introduce our friend to Jesus and explain his concerns. Then one could say that we have led our friend to Jesus. We know if this were possible, Jesus would hold His hand out to our friend. If our friend takes His hand, Jesus will not only give him the right to become God's child **(John 1:12-13)**, Jesus will also give your friend's weary soul His strength, peace, and direction **(Matthew 11:28-30)**.

By faith, we helpers know that Jesus is near and we can take the seeker by the hand (in prayer) and Jesus will offer His hand of grace. The way a seeker, saved or unsaved, takes Jesus' hand is in accepting His word. When Jesus gives a word of instruction, comfort or understanding, the acceptance of that word is taking His hand. We know this because we too are seekers along the narrow path who realize we cannot travel very far without Jesus. All of us are subject to straying from the path and getting overwhelmed and even lost in the darkness. Taking Jesus' hand is our daily exercise of faith. Sometimes we can get so discouraged in the midst of the darkness, we need a friend to help us find our way to Jesus.

When visiting one-to-one with a friend at the nursing home or sharing the message in a church service, one important goal is to encourage your friends to take Jesus' hand so that He can lead them along the narrow path. If they reach out to Jesus, He is faithful to take their hand and walk with them in their valley. The way to do this is to respectfully share a fresh, down-to-earth perspective of Jesus' way, His love, or one of His promises. As they accept God's Word, agree with them in prayer for its fulfillment in their lives. Accepting God's word will often include letting go of past beliefs, sins or even grudges toward others. We must be patient and prayerful as this may take more than a few visits.

Jesus said; "Come to me, all you who are weary and burdened, and I will give you rest. Take my yoke upon you and learn from me, for I am gentle and humble in heart, and you will find rest for your souls. For my yoke is easy and my burden is light" (Matthew 11:27-30).

Sinner's Prayers

Last week, at the nursing home, I (Bill) shared with residents how, over twenty years ago, a friend of mine encouraged me to pray a special prayer. I further explained that this prayer was the first step I took that had greatly changed my life and made me what I am today. I also shared some Scriptures and told them how important it was to invite Jesus into our heart and to accept Him as Lord and Savior. As the church service came to a close, we passed a copy of the prayer to those in attendance (about 45). I first read it aloud, then asked if they would like to pray this prayer with me. I explained that the LORD Jesus would answer, if they prayed from their heart. So we began to pray slowly. I watched with great encouragement as most of the residents prayed. After the prayer, I asked, "Did you pray this prayer?" If so, would you publicly express your decision by lifting your paper up above your head?" About 90% of the audience, including a staff person and a family member raised their prayers up with smiles. Then we sang the chorus, "He is LORD."

After the service, my wife and I shared a copy of the prayer with several individuals who also prayed and received Jesus into their hearts. What a joyful day this was for many!

In the same way, I tell you, there is rejoicing in the presence of the angels of God over one sinner who repents (Luke 15:10).

A traditional sinner's prayer would be:
Lord Jesus, I know that I am a sinner and need your forgiveness. I believe that you died on the cross for the sins of all people including mine. I purpose to turn from all my sins and I invite you to come into my heart to live in me and guide my life. I desire to trust you as my Lord and Savior all the days of my life. Amen.

Another example of a sinner's prayer is:
Father God, I ask that you would receive me as your child. I come to you because I believe that Jesus made forgiveness of my sins possible through His death on the cross and his resurrection from the dead. I ask that you would have mercy on me and accept me as your child and servant forever. I ask this in the name of Jesus Christ my Lord and Savior. Amen.

These kinds of prayers have been used in many different situations in the past and have been the beginning of life in Christ for millions of repentant sinners. If you are able to help your friends pray like this from their heart, you can be sure that our merciful Father in Heaven has accepted them. However, a person's mental and physical state may not afford them the ability to articulate so many words. It is important, therefore, to realize that such a traditional sinner's prayer is not a specific command in the Bible for salvation. The Bible is clear that a person must believe enough to put his trust in Jesus. There are many examples in the Bible of sinners who cried out to the Lord and received His grace:

- A man with leprosy; Mark 1:40-44
- The Sinner's cry: "If you are willing, you can make me clean."
- Jesus' response: "I am willing. Be clean."
- A blind man; Mark 10:46-52
- The Sinner's cry: "Jesus, Son of David, have mercy on me!"
- Jesus' response: "What do you want me to do for you?"
- The sinner's request: "Rabbi, I want to see."
- Jesus' response: "Go," said Jesus, "your faith has healed you."
- A lost son (parable); Luke 15:11-32
- The sinner's cry: "Father, I have sinned against heaven and against you. I am no longer worthy to be called your son."

The father's response: "Quick! Bring the best robe and put it on him. Put a ring on his finger and sandals on his feet. Bring the fattened calf and kill it. Let's have a feast and celebrate. For this son of mine was dead and is alive again; he was lost and is found."

- Ten lepers; Luke 17:11-19
- The sinner's cry: "Jesus, Master, have pity on us!"
- Jesus' reply: "Go show yourselves to the priests." "Rise and go, your faith has made you well."
- A tax collector, (parable); Luke 18:9-14
- The sinner's cry: "God, have mercy on me, a sinner."
- Jesus' reply: "I tell you that this man…went home justified before God."
- A man on the cross next to Jesus; Luke 23:40-43

- The sinner's cry: "Jesus, remember me when you come into your kingdom."
- Jesus' response: "I tell you the truth, today you will be with me in paradise."
- A thief; Luke 19:1-10
- The sinner's confession: "Look, Lord! Here and now I give half of my possessions to the poor, and if I have cheated anybody out of anything, I will pay back four times the amount."
- Jesus' response: "Today salvation has come to this house."

> One week when we were conducting a service on the Alzheimer's Unit, I asked if anyone knew the first song we usually sing. (It's always the same song.) No one answered. We proceeded to play the music from the same tape that we use every week. I always tell our friends that they are doing a very important thing--praising Jesus our LORD and Savior and praying for others. I also tell them, before the last song we sing, "God Bless America," we are praying for all the people in this country.
>
> At the end of our time together, a resident in the group shouted "I HAVE DECIDED TO FOLLOW JESUS!" That was our first song. We all praised God and applauded. It was a wonderful time. But the next week when we came back, we discovered this woman had died. She had done what she had confessed, and truly followed Jesus.
>
> Mary Ann Goodrich

Would this woman's prayer be less received by our merciful Savior than any other sincere sinner's prayer? We need to keep in mind: Whenever a humble sinner cried out to the Lord, whatever his situation, the Lord answered his cry. This is the grace of God. God required no one specific prayer and demanded or expected no one specific response. Peter said, **"Everyone who calls on the name of the Lord will be saved" (Acts 2:21).** And we are reminded in **2 Samuel 1:4** that *God devises ways so that a banished person may not remain estranged from him.*

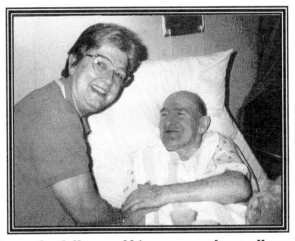

From the fullness of his grace we have all received one blessing after another. For the law was given through Moses; grace and truth came through Jesus Christ (John 1:16-17).

CHAPTER 6

CARE TEAMS AND GROUP SERVICES

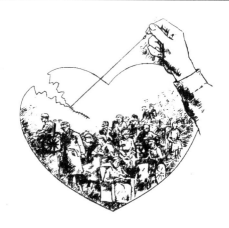

> *"Many care-facility residents feel deeply the need for gathering with other believers in a fashion similar to the memories they hold dear from their experiences in their home church. They want to sing the old hymns and choruses they learned years ago. They want someone to pray with them for their needs and concerns. They want someone to share with them encouragement and exhortation from God's Word."*
>
> Gerald & Dar Johnson,
> *A Handbook for Nursing Home Ministry*

When visiting one-to-one in a nursing home, individuals or teams of two people can accomplish desired goals. When a church decides to provide a group service, a larger, more structured team is recommended for maximum effectiveness. Many churches desire to conduct a group service and begin such a ministry with good intentions, but soon fizzle out for a number of reasons:

1. Team members quit because they feel inadequate or that they are not being useful.
2. The team feels it is not being effective due to lack of positive response from the residents.
3. The team runs into problems it does not know how to handle.
4. Team members do not receive support from their church leadership.
5. The inherent difficulties and challenges of nursing home-ministry discourage the team.

Having a structured team and following the guidelines outlined in this book will greatly assist you and minimize these concerns.

THE MINISTRY CARE TEAM'S ROLE

Although a large number of volunteers can make up a care team for group services, it is normally made up of four to six Christians. There are four different positions that make up a Ministry Care Team. Below are brief descriptions for each position. Following the descriptions, we have included some specific details on how the team can work together to provide a quality Christ-centered worship service. It is common for a person to take on more than one of these care team positions, but each team member should be given an opportunity to exercise and develop personal gifts and skills. The positions are as follows:

- **Team Coordinator:** This person keeps the team together by communicating with team members, praying with and for the team members, and coordinating an occasional team fellowship hour to encourage and strengthen members. This person is also the one who would maintain any needed records and also be the communication link between team members, the Activities Director and the home-church leadership.

- **Teacher:** This person is responsible to prayerfully prepare a message for the church service/Bible study. In either case, the message generally follows a time of worship, praise and prayer.

- **Song Leader**: This person is responsible to prepare for and lead group singing. This usually takes about twenty minutes at the beginning of a group service. The song leader can lead using an instrument or special accompanying CD's and large print hymnals designed for nursing home ministry. (See our Resource Chapter).

- Sometimes two individuals share this responsibility, one playing the instrument while the other is the more visible song leader.

- **Helpers:** These people are responsible to help other team members accomplish their tasks. Helpers also help bring residents to church services, assist residents with turning pages of their hymn books, take attendance, etc. The helpers' role on the Ministry Care Team is **very important** because they help the services flow smoothly. Many shy people start out as helpers. After several months of involvement, they might move into other team positions, and find themselves blossoming in their additional giftings.

John is more than a helper. He's a very busy and important man to the large corporation where he works. When he can, he takes time to come a long way to see the people at the nursing home and help them get to the church service. He is so cheerful and kind, they all love him and he loves them.

One week, after being touched by a Christmas message, "Jesus is the Light of the World," John decided to make the residents a present. He made 50 freestanding plaques of wood, routed the edges, painted the name of JESUS in gold and put a gold painted Christmas tree light on top of each one. I can't even imagine how many hours of work and love went into them.

Many of the residents put the plaques on top of their TV's. Now, a few years later, I go into the rooms and still see the name of JESUS shining in gold on top of some TV's. I praise the Lord over and over. Every nurse, caregiver, family member, and doctor who enters that room sees the name of JESUS more prominently than anything else. What a continued blessing for all of us. Thank you, John.

Mary Ann Goodrich

All team members have a common goal: to prayerfully enable an opportunity for all willing residents to worship the Lord and grow in understanding His Word through Christ-centered services. Through personal relationships with residents and staff, our message finds its platform. Faithful and consistent visits have proven to be the best way to establish this platform.

We recommend that your team focus on only one nursing home in your church's community, and that you make it your goal to visit on a weekly basis. If the team grows to eight or more consistent team members, a second team could be established to adopt another nursing home in the community. This second team will function independently but the two teams should come together periodically for fellowship, encouragement (perhaps at a luncheon meeting), and prayer support.

It is very normal for your church service or Bible study to start out with only five or ten residents. However, once the word gets around that the services are a blessing, it is common for your group to grow to include up to fifty percent or more of the nursing home's population.

WORSHIP SERVICES

We pray in the opening of each church service we conduct in care facilities. This is formally called an invocation. At the end of each church service we also pray. This is formally called a benediction, in which we again ask the Lord to touch and strengthen hearts and thank Him for the blessings we have received. In our prayers, we often ask the Lord to forgive us of our sins, to lift suffering off those who are hurting and to save the souls of those we each may know who are lost. We consider these prayers to be vital "bookends" to our efforts.

On occasion, it is obviously appropriate to pray in the middle of the service. This prayer may be a way to draw the audience back into a worshipful attitude after some disruption or distraction. Or, we may pray for specific needs that we are aware of in our group. In some cases, residents will pass along to us prayer requests and the names of those in the hospital or those very ill and in bed.

At some point in our prayers, during the service, we are careful to pray for the staff of the facility and for the residents who were not able to make it to the service. God is good, and He gracefully responds to the prayerful faith in our cry, and the faith in the hearts of our audience, for His intervention on their behalf.

Gerald & Dar Johnson,
A Handbook for Nursing Home Ministry

There are several models for worship services. We have outlined two that have been used over the years. We recommend you begin by using a time proven model, and then make adjustments as you see the need. Remember, it takes time to develop a quality service, and mistakes are part of the learning process. Be open for correction, make necessary adjustments, and you will see the glory of God.

SUGGESTED MODEL FOR WORSHIP SERVICES (TRADITIONAL)

This model is a somewhat traditional form chosen to match the expectations of the wide variety of traditions and experiences represented by nursing home residents, and to adjust to the unique particulars of the nursing home situation. (Total time: 30-45 minutes)

We have found it beneficial to announce at the beginning of the service that we are willing to talk or pray with individuals after the service. Those who have a desire to share their extensive needs and deeply felt emotions during the service will then be satisfied to wait. After the service we ask those who desire prayer, or who may just want to talk, to raise their hands.

Introduction

Introduce yourself and any new team members, and welcome all in attendance. This time is normally more casual in nature and may include announcements, song requests for the service and a little levity. Take the time to express appreciation to the residents for allowing you to be with them in their home, assuring them how you consider this time together and in the presence of our Lord a great privilege and honor.

Call to Worship

A psalm (such as **Psalm 95 or 100**) is useful here, read clearly and slowly.

Invocation

Your opening prayer should be clear, authoritative, and brief.

Songs

Singing brings involvement and awakens past experiences of worship. Large print hymnals with familiar hymns should be used. Requests for favorites songs can be an added blessing (we recommend requests be shared before the call to worship to prevent the worship service from being choppy).

Scripture

Scripture may be read at this point or during your message. Many teams take a few minutes in this part of the service for Scripture memorization. A good Scripture portion to recite together from memory is **Psalm 23**. This Psalm is very dear to many, was often learned early in life, and is full of truth, beauty and comfort. The exercise of reciting from memory also stimulates the mind and heart and can give a sense of achievement.

Message

A message or sermon ten to fifteen minutes in length should be sufficient. Make a very few basic points (even just one), freely use illustrations or stories which relate to the residents, and apply to the message and Scripture used. End the message with a clear, encouraging challenge.

Prayer

The prayer can be either a corporate prayer or a prayer by the leader. Remember, too, that much training in intercession can be done by example. Many teams close the prayer by reciting together the Lord's Prayer. **(Matthew 6:9-13)**

Closing Song

Depending on the time available and alertness or eagerness of the residents, a closing song related to the message may help to seal the message in their hearts.

Closing

Close with a brief scriptural blessing (e.g., **Jude 24-25; Hebrews 13:20-21; 2Corinthians 13:14; Numbers 6:24-26**; and/or the singing of the **Doxology**).

SUGGESTED MODEL FOR WORSHIP SERVICES (CASUAL)

> *"When we sing, we do so with much **feeling** and **enthusiasm** and **energy**. We do everything we can to encourage the residents to sing with us and clap their hands to the faster tunes if they are able and are so inclined. Often, we comment on the songs, before or after singing them, regarding their message and their relevance to them in their situation. As often as possible, we try to tie together our sermonette with the message in the song on the tape that we use to precede or follow it."*
>
> Gerald & Dar Johnson,
> *A Handbook for Nursing Home Ministry*

This suggested model for worship uses stories throughout the service. It is as if the message were presented in short portions, spread out over the whole service, rather than given in a separate 10-15 minute segment. Based on a text and/or a topic from a text; like *contentment* or *forgiveness*, find three or four short stories or illustrations. Books of illustrations (or often websites) are very useful here, as are other sources, for example emails from friends or magazines like *Guideposts* or *The Reader's Digest*. Nursing home residents, like most of us, enjoy stories and usually eagerly pay attention to a good one. By the time we finish, we've heard some good stories, we've talked about the biblical point of the stories using Scripture, we've sung songs related to the topic, we've prayed about the topic as it relates to our lives, and we have given our lives afresh to God, asking for His help in our circumstances and thanking Him for His mercy and kindness. The model, which follows, is one combination of these elements. (Total time: 30-45 minutes).

Introduction

It is beneficial to express gratitude for how God allows all of us from different churches and cultures to come together to worship Jesus.

Opening Psalm

Usually just a few verses from a Psalm, for example **Psalm 92, 95, 96,** or **100.**

Opening Prayer

Thank God for who He is and what He has done; welcome His presence.

Hymn #1 & #2

Story #1

This first story will introduce the theme chosen for the service.

Hymn #3

This hymn is usually directly related to the theme.

Story #2

This story could be shared by a different team member.

Special music, poem or prayer

This also could be shared by a different team member.

Scripture Reading and Summary

This message brings all the stories and the Scripture together usually challenging the audience to embrace the Scriptural point of the theme, (usually only 5-7 minutes).

Hymn #4

Hymn #5 (if time, often a request)

Closing Prayer
This prayer includes a corporate confession of faith or acceptance of the challenge shared throughout the theme.

SUGGESTED MODEL FOR A BIBLE STUDY

Bible studies are very similar to the above church services. The primary difference is that there is usually more group interaction. One person says, *"Generally,* s*ermons are given; Bible studies are shared."* Bible studies are usually more informal, allowing residents an opportunity to share experiences and insights from Scripture, and to ask questions. Christian bookstores always have many different Bible study guides that can be used for ministry with a variety of formats. Most include guidelines for leaders on how to conduct a group study. Many are based on themes that would be appropriate for nursing homes (for example loneliness, hope, facing death and the future life). Some leaders prefer to teach on a passage of Scripture; others prefer a more inductive approach that includes reading a passage of Scripture and asking questions (Total time: 30-45 minutes).

Introduction

As noted in the worship service models, it is beneficial to express gratitude for how God allows all of us from different churches and cultures to come together to worship Him and study His word. You can say to the group, "The reason we can all be together like this is because we are all here to seek, love, and know the same Person, the central Person of all our Christian denominations, Jesus Christ." This kind of proclamation is powerful in helping residents recognize the difference between a relationship with Jesus and a particular denomination or religion.

Opening prayer

Encourage prayer requests from residents. After all requests are spoken, the leader can pray for each request and also ask the Lord to bless the staff, residents, residents' families and the service.

Songs

Some Bible studies incorporate about five songs; others do not sing any songs. Note that in the Bible study service, songs may include less traditional ones in addition to those in the hymnbook. Residents may enjoy learning some new hymns and choruses, especially if they are sung every week and can be memorized.

Transition

After the last song, the team collects the songbooks and/or hymnbooks and passes out the Scripture portions that are printed in Large Print and copied *for all to keep*. (See appendix for a few examples of large-print Scripture papers.) Music is played in the background during this transition.

Message

The teacher may invite residents to read along with all or part of the Scripture on the paper. Then the teacher will share the message or use the Scripture to raise questions and engage the residents in discussion. Scripture memorization may be included with the Bible study. Residents usually enjoy an inductive Bible Study approach, giving them an opportunity to share their thoughts on Scripture.

Closing prayer

The teacher or other team member will lead the group in a prayer for receiving the principles and instruction, etc., shared throughout the message. A closing song can also be sung.

In the next chapter, we will offer you many more guidelines for group ministry in the nursing home. You will also find an abundance of resources in our Resource Chapter.

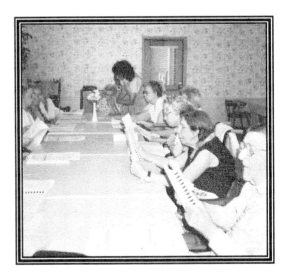

Give us each day our daily bread (Luke 11:3).

CHAPTER 7

TIPS FOR EFFECTIVE GROUP MINISTRY

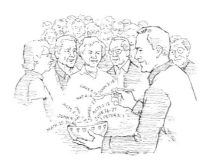

It is a good idea for the ministry team members to ask each other; "How can we help the Christians in the nursing home live out the remainder of their lives in such a way that the Lord will say at their entry, 'Well done!'" Below is a more detailed list of tips and guidelines that will assist team members in adding quality to the services, while anticipating and removing as many distractions as possible. Do not allow yourself to become overwhelmed by the many points shared here; look through them and consider ones that would be most helpful.

Before you enter the home:

- It's a good idea for the team to meet fifteen minutes to a half-hour before going to the nursing home so members can share in fellowship and prayer. This time will allow all team members to share and pray over personal issues so that they can better focus on the residents' needs when arriving at the home.

- Leave your denomination at your church. Lift Jesus up! Preach Christ! (See information on overcoming denominational walls in Chapter Five.)

- Have a specific plan, but always be prepared for the unexpected. Sometimes the unexpected is the Lord's perfect plan.

Room set-up:

- Move the furniture, if appropriate. The less cluttered the room, the less distracting and the more pleasant the environment.
- Have your song leader play meditative music while the residents are being gathered. We recommend you begin by playing the music softly, at about 1/2 the volume that you will be using during the service. After a few minutes turn it up to about 3/4 volume. This allows for a slow and more welcomed change in the community room.
- If there is a television on in the room which you will not be using, be sensitive to those who are watching. Here is a suggestion we have found works well: After the room is set up and the music is playing, ask residents/staff for permission to turn the TV off. It is helpful to first invite the individuals watching the TV to the service before shutting it off. Residents are less resistant to turning the TV off when they hear the music in the background. If there is ever a problem with turning the TV off, talk with the Activities Director about a remedy.

I (Bill) often have people say to me that they do not need a microphone because they can project their voice well. I, too, have a strong and fairly deep voice. I spent my first seven years ministering without a sound system. I was very surprised at the difference even a low-cost system made for the residents. I have demonstrated this fact with ease during our training workshops. After using my portable sound system for about half of the day, I turn it off for a few minutes to show the audience the difference. There are no questions about its effectiveness after that. We have also found that many people have a natural tendency to sound angry when trying to speak loudly. Using a microphone alleviates this problem. If you do not use a microphone, be aware of how you sound to others. Ask for honest feedback from your audience.

Notes on sound systems and their use:

Although some of us have a strong speaking voice, we still recommend the use of a quality sound system to project the sound of your voice. There are many options available on the market that range in price and quality. You will want your system to be lightweight and portable, as well as easy to set up. A sound system can be somewhat expensive, so shop around for the best buy. Below is a list of things to consider:

- Quality and easy transportability does make a big difference.

- Systems that have at least a 15-watt output normally have acceptable sound quality. We recommend you do not waste your money on one that is lower than 7 watts, or one that is excessively powerful.

- Systems with an equalizer allow for the best sound control.

- Some audio stores sell a portable microphone that will broadcast over an FM band. This would allow you to use a portable boom box that does not have a microphone jack. Note: This is only useful for speaking through the FM radio band and cannot be used at the same time that the CD or cassette player is playing.

- A bargain-priced microphone can distort the sound of a quality amplifier. It is usually better to spend the extra few dollars on a better one if you possibly can. Be sure to test the sound quality before you purchase any equipment.

- Remember, audio stores normally have very good acoustics so your system may sound different in the nursing home.

- Having two speakers that are detachable and can be placed a few inches higher than the residents' heads will project the sound across the room much better than a unit that is set up on the floor. If the system is lower than the residents' heads, the folks in the front will get most of the sound while the folks in the back will get the muffled leftovers.

- If possible, place the speakers ten to fifteen feet apart and pointing toward the center of the back of the room. This helps to spread the sound evenly.

- The terrible shriek sound that comes out of the speakers is called feedback. It is usually caused if the microphone is put too close or in front of a speaker. Lowering the main volume or repositioning the microphone behind the speakers will help. A unidirectional microphone is another recommendation for limiting feedback.

- If you plan to use Sing-a-long tapes or CD's to accompany you, you must plan accordingly. In our experience, CD's have proved to be more practical and user friendly than the tapes, because the CD allows jumping immediately to a selected song, which you frequently want to do, especially when allowing for resident requests.

- Consider inviting your church to take up a special offering to cover the costs of equipment. This is a good opportunity to allow the whole congregation to be a support and blessing to the nursing home. Some teams have been successful in raising the needed funds by dividing the total cost of the equipment by the number of families in their church, then asking the pastor to encourage a special offering from each family. The amount needed is usually less than $10 per family.

- Because you will need to transfer the sound system from your home to the nursing home on a weekly basis, an extended warranty is recommended in case damage occurs during transport.

Gathering the residents:

- Offer to help the staff bring residents to the service. This is often a welcomed support for the nursing and activities departments, and will allow you to gather more residents in a shorter time. This is also a great time of fellowship while wheeling friends to and from the service, as well as an opportunity to pray for specific concerns. As you walk through the halls, you will likely encounter residents who may not be able to come to the service that day but would appreciate a short prayer. Occasionally, the activities director will not permit volunteers to bring residents to the church service. The primary reason for this is that they may have had a bad experience with residents being pressured into going to the church service. Be patient; as trusting relationships are built with the staff, more freedom will be given to you. Remember not to give any physical care to a resident; if they need to be transferred from a bed to a wheelchair, for example, ask help from the nursing staff.

- Never force residents to go to the service. Sometimes, well-meaning volunteers believe that if they can just get someone into the service, the Lord will help them more. Although this thought is well intentioned and may be true, for many reasons we find the following approach to be more appropriate and effective. While positioning yourself at eye level, and offering a gentle hand-shake, say and do something like the following:
    - "Hi Miss Jones, How are you doing today?"
    - Give her a moment to reply.

- ➢ "We are having a Bible study (or church service) in a few moments in the dinning room tonight. Would you like to join us?"
- ➢ She may ask what church you are from.
- ➢ You can say, "I attend ____ but everyone is welcome to attend this Bible study; we sing some of the old hymns, read from the Bible to learn more about Jesus, and pray together."
- ➢ If she says "No," just politely say, "OK, maybe next time" or "OK, but if you ever want to join us, you are more than welcome."
- ➢ This response gives the resident the opportunity to make a personal choice; a rare experience in an institutionalized setting. We have experienced many residents, who after saying "No," later change their mind, possibly because of the freedom to choose.
- ➢ Your invitation should not be rushed. However, be careful not to take too long, because likely there are many more to be gathered for the service. If you sense the need to spend more time, you could say, "I have many other folks to help get to the service. May I come back to see you after the service?" If they agree, please do not forget to return.
- ➢ Ending this encounter with a kind word or "God bless you" is normally well received.
- If possible, position residents close together in a semi-circle, leaving enough space for the helpers to walk between the rows for assisting residents.
- Arrange people in the room in such a fashion that if someone in the middle needs to leave during the service, the disruption would be minimal.
- Some folks can unintentionally (and sometimes intentionally) create disturbances. Gather these friends

who may interrupt the service last. Seating them in the front just prior to the start of the service helps to keep them attentive and quiet. It also allows them to leave or be taken out if that becomes necessary. Exactly where you seat them may vary depending on where the room exit is. Be sure and have helpers who are free to move people in and out of a service.

- There are a few hearing-impaired residents in every group. Find a special place with their hearing ear positioned near one of the speakers. They appreciate this!

- Maintain an attendance roster whenever possible. This will help you to remember new folks and remind you of ones that may need a personal visit. Most nursing homes require attendance at all activities, so this can be a help to the staff as well.

Praise & worship time:

- The old hymns and choruses are what most Christian residents in nursing homes have grown up with. Please be careful not to impose on them your own preferred style of music that may seem more upbeat but would not be familiar. Remember, although you may not appreciate the old styles, the residents usually love them and we are there to bless our friends, not ourselves. You will find that the old hymns have a lot to offer all of us...and they do grow on you.

- Residents can more easily participate in the singing when the music is played at a lower key and at a slower-than-usual tempo. (Not all pianists can easily make this adjustment, but do your best to accommodate.)

- Speak LOUDLY, slooowly, and clearly when introducing songs. Repeat the number and give ample time for residents to find their page by playing through the song at least one time before you sing it. Assist only those who need the help.

> *One very helpful practice is to announce to the audience what you are going to do before you do it.*
> *Examples: "Now I would like to read a portion of Scripture... Now, we are going to have Joe come up to share in a time of prayer with us".*
> *This practice has really helped to keep the not-so-alert residents in the flow of the service.*

- Avoid introducing too many new songs. People like new songs, but do limit them to one or two in a service. Some newer songs or choruses can be effectively used as special music presented by the care team; often well-chosen songs allow and invite group participation.
- Some teams have experimented with using songs (in large and bold print) on an overhead, projected onto a wall or screen. This works well for some, eliminating the problems of handling a song book and giving more freedom to choose a wider variety of songs than often found in large print hymnals. Do not assume, however, that this technique will work in the home in which you minister in; space, lighting and resident preferences all must be considered.

The message:

- Be sure you have a point to make in your message. Keep the message uncluttered with many details and stick to your point. Remember, every message should encourage all to trust Jesus.
- Use stories and illustrations to flavor your message and help people relate to the Biblical truths presented.
- A 10 or 15 minute message is often received and appreciated more than a 30-45 minute message.
- Avoid preaching on topics that have little meaning to people who are in their later years, like your opinions, controversial denominational differences or discouraging

current events. Instead, focus on the practical application of biblical truths for living today.

- Avoid preaching against the religious practices of others. Lift up what is *right* rather than focusing on what is *wrong*.
- One of the areas you will be teaching/preaching on is salvation. Remember that there are other spiritual needs that nursing home residents have, for example, hope, love, peace and faith. There are countless messages in the Bible to help encourage the fulfillment of these spiritual needs. Consider also examples and illustrations found in daily devotionals such as *Our Daily Bread, The Upper Room, Strength and Peace.* (See our Resource Chapter).
- Encourage residents' involvement with the message. Some teachers type the Scripture verses in large print and give them to the residents. While sharing the message, they may have people repeat certain verses or even adjectives like *all, every, whosoever*. These words help them to realize that they, personally, are included in God's plans and promises. Large print Bibles are also welcome additions for residents who can hold them. Your church might also be interested in purchasing these for a home.

Closing the message:

- Don't be afraid to challenge the residents, but do not pressure or intimidate them; rather, be gentle, clear and gracious.
- One of the appreciated skills of a preacher/teacher is knowing when to stop.
- Seal the message with prayer. Ask the Lord to give us all "good and believing hearts" so that the seeds of His Word might bear much fruit. (See **Matthew 13:10-23**)
- One of the main goals in the teaching or preaching in a group service is to help the hearers gain a fresh perspective on the person of Jesus Christ, such as His love, His faithfulness, His willingness to forgive, help, and guide, etc.

Once people gain this perspective, the teacher can then encourage and challenge them to take steps of faith to draw near to Him. These steps always start with a prayer of acceptance of the Word that was just shared.

The Closing Prayer:

There are many ways to close a service with prayer:
- The leader can take requests and then offer them to the Lord for the group.
- The leader leads all in a prayer by saying one phrase at a time and the rest repeat it.
- A prayer is written out on the program that pertains to the message and all are encouraged to pray the prayer together.
- The Lord's Prayer can be prayed in unison after the leader's prayer.
- Songs are a way of singing a prayer. Good examples are: Just a Closer Walk With Thee, He is Lord, Just as I Am, Great is Thy Faithfulness, and God Bless America.

Before you leave:

- As many team members as possible, but at least the preacher/teacher, should shake hands with all residents before the residents disperse. Team members also can be available to offer individual prayer for those who desire it.
- If you are responsible for helping residents return to their rooms, be sure that their call light is within reaching distance before you leave the room. This is also a good time to ask them how you can pray for them, and then pray before you leave the room.
- Leave the meeting room in order and cleaner than when you found it.

Other tips:

- Evaluate your team's effectiveness. Consider the questions at the end of this chapter

- Every ministry is challenged with problems. Praying for wisdom to overcome problems is often more effective than praying for problems to go away.
- The worship service/Bible study that you share in a nursing home may be quite different from the one you have at your church; however, they should be of no lesser quality.

A couple of years ago my husband and I got involved with nursing home ministry through our church. We went to several different homes. Some every other week, some once a month. If there was a holiday the residents were the ones who missed out, due to whatever the coordinator scheduled. A friend of ours convinced us to attend a training program and purchase some of the music and songbooks displayed there. Well, I have to admit it has all been a great hit.

We started all over again, using suggestions we learned in the training class – we decided to focus on one nursing home out of the several that our church was visiting. The people in the home said, "Two weeks was too long to go without hearing God's Word," so we now meet weekly to share in a Bible study.

We have seen such a change in the friends we now have. Where before we always got the same blank stares; now we have a group of people who are not only prayer warriors, but are concerned about each other. Through these techniques and supplies, we now have a group of caring, living, loving friends. Before, they just existed in their own little world, almost afraid to love or be loved. It has taken time, patience, and a lot of work to have such great results, but we see our labor is not in vain.   Pat Mathena

SOME GUIDELINES FOR THE TEACHER

*Those who are seekers and followers of Jesus have the same desire as the Greeks in **John 12:20-21**. Their request was, **"Sir, we wish to see Jesus."***

*The minister's desire should be like that of John the Baptist who said, **"He must increase, I must decrease" (John 3:30)**. The more we decrease, the more Christ will increase in our ministry. And as we lift up the name of Jesus, all men will be drawn to Him **(John 12:32)**.*

We find it important that the teacher, i.e. the person delivering the sermon or leading the Bible study, have a proper perspective in regard to his role. When this perspective is based on Biblical principles, there is great potential for being very effective. Below are a few points to consider:

- Never forget who you are as a servant of the Lord. He uses you as a teacher to share His Word. Teachers are also co-laborers with the rest of the team; you should be one body held together with cords of love. If you become successful and favored by your hearers, rejoice, but don't become proud (**Proverbs 18:12** and **James 4:6).**

- The Word of God is best shared in the love of God. *"Speak the truth in love" (Eph. 4:15)*. An abundance of love without a good portion of truth can lead to a watered-down message, resulting in a superficial hope. On the other hand, an abundance of the Word without a good measure of love can misrepresent the gracious character of the Lord.

There can be great joy in seeing an elderly person not only confess faith in Jesus with the words of their mouth, but also grow in that faith. This is the desired fruit of our labors. Our experience is that this may come at a slower pace than what we may sometimes desire. Each message shared is like adding a few drops of food coloring to a large tank of water. Each individual drop appears to have little effect. However, each individual drop adds to the others and in time, change will be obvious. Waiting for faith to grow can also be compared to watching a tree grow. The growth is slow enough to discourage any impatient viewer, but the faithful and consistent gardener will one day enjoy its fruit.

Message preparation:

- Prayer is essential for your preparation. During the week, ask the Lord to teach you what to share with His people in the nursing home. You will likely learn much more in your studies than you can share in one service. Be sensitive. Don't overwhelm your audience. It is also a great help to have other Christians interceding for you.

- Before putting the message together, ask yourself what the major point will be. This is sometimes the most difficult part of preparing the message.

- Alternating through the different focuses of the residents' spiritual needs will help make your messages interesting and keep you from concentrating too much in one area. Preaching weekly through a larger Scripture portion can both help guide you and direct you to cover many areas of concern. Some suggested passages are Psalm 23, The Beatitudes, The Lord's Prayer, or a gospel such as the book of John; each meeting's portion should be appropriately "bite-sized."

- Whatever your main point, it should be relevant to today's concerns, and encourage trust, hope, and submission to our Lord Jesus.

- The best Bible teachers study their Bible on a regular basis and know how to break down their learning into understandable points so that all may receive.

- Use a concordance as you prepare. Find as many Scriptures as you need to specifically address your main point. This will help you gain a deeper understanding of your focus. Plan, however, to share only three or four of these Scriptures so that the message is not overbearing or too long. Avoid Scripture-hopping. Keep the message clear.

- Reading from several translations of the Bible will help you gain a deeper and more balanced understanding of the Word. Older people may prefer to hear or read from an older familiar translation such as the King James version. However, a translation in today's language is much easier to understand.

- Plan to share from your heart so that the message flows smoothly and is not choppy. Using an outline rather than reading your message may aid in this.

- Writing passages of Scripture on paper is very helpful for the residents to follow and read along. (18-point type in **"Times New Roman Bold"** or **"Arial Black"** font is readable by most residents.)

- Write out a short prayer on the bottom of the paper that will help the congregation or study group understand and embrace the point of your message. As mentioned in Chapter 5, when people accept the Lord's Word, they are accepting the Lord. Your closing prayer can assist your audience in expressing their acceptance.

- Consider questions you can ask during a church service or Bible study that residents might enjoy responding to with brief answers.

- Pray and seek a mentor with whom you can share/practice your message in order to obtain honest feedback.

THREE PARTS OF A TOPICAL SERMON

The following is a suggested outline for sermon preparation:

1. **Beginning** – What is the Issue/Concern/Problem?
2. **Middle** – Biblical example of #1, and how Jesus intervened
3. **End** - Application; How do #1 & #2 relate to us today? It is helpful to include an illustration or a personal testimony related to your main point.

   Main Point:

   A) Challenge; What is the Lord saying to us personally?
      - a sin I should keep away from?
      - a promise I can call my own?
      - a command for me to obey?
      - a blessing I can enjoy?
      - a failure from which I can learn?
      - a victory for me to win?
      - a new thought about God, the Lord Jesus, the Holy Spirit, Satan, people?
      - a truth in this passage that has greatly affected me?

   B) Prayer; of accepting the word and intervention of Jesus in our lives.

THREE PARTS OF A BIBLE STUDY

The following outline for a Bible study or devotional is very similar. The difference is that your beginning will be a specific Scripture portion:

Main Point
1. **Beginning** – Scripture portion/story/event/parable
2. **Middle** – Basic explanation of #1, focusing on the intervention of the Lord and any related scriptures
3. **End** – Application; Challenge; Prayer of acceptance

Parts 2 & 3 are the main points of your sermon or Bible study. Your main point needs to be focused on an attribute or action of Jesus Christ. For example, His:

Love	Suffering
Promises	Faithfulness
Willingness to help	Will & Commands
Relationship with the Father	Presence
Power & Authority	The Kingdom of Heaven

GROUP-MINISTRY EVALUATION

An essential component to encouraging and keeping your care team together is to occasionally gather for a time of communication and evaluation of your ministry and its effectiveness. We recommend the setting to be casual, perhaps over a meal. Below is a list of questions that can be asked. Care must be exercised to offer much encouragement and appreciation for those who have been faithful to the mission. Do not be hard on yourselves as you ask these questions. The purpose for this gathering is not to criticize, but to critique. This critique should improve your effectiveness and increase your joy. Also, be sure to give each member an opportunity to share a blessing about their visits and to discuss areas of possible improvement.

- Did we encourage the residents?
- Did we challenge them to take steps of faith closer to Jesus?

- Did we help them with prayer?
- Did we offend anyone?
- Is the primary topic of our messages focused on Jesus?
- Do all the residents come to the services/study who want to come?
- Do the services flow or are they choppy?
- Does every resident receive a greeting from at least one team member?
- Do we thank the Lord for answering our prayer for help?
- What one or two things could we do to improve our effectiveness?
- How can we better help our friends live out the remainder of their lives in such a way that the Lord will say at their face-to-face meeting with Him, "Well done!"

As we faithfully study and share the Word of God, the Lord opens amazing truths to us that can impact our own lives as well as the lives of our hearers. These truths are often hidden from the casual observer, but as we apply the principles which we learn, they become our eternal blessings. What an awesome privilege to possess and share these heavenly treasures through Christ Jesus our Lord.

> *No eye has seen, no ear has heard, no mind has conceived what God has prepared for those who love Him—but God has revealed it to us by His Spirit.*
>
> **1 Corinthians 2:9-10**

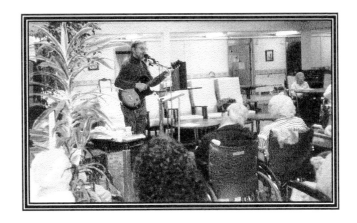

Man does not live on bread alone, but on every word that comes from the mouth of God (Matthew 4:4).

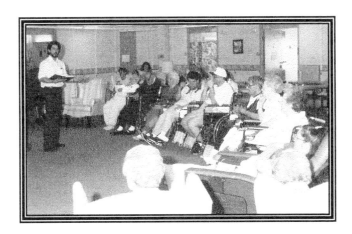

God is not unjust; he will not forget your work and the love you have shown him as you have helped his people and continue to help them (Hebrews 6:10)

CHAPTER 8

MINISTERING BEYOND THE LIMITATIONS OF DEMENTIA

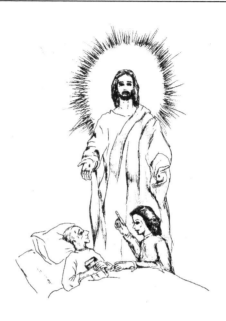

So we fix our eyes not on what is seen, but on what is unseen. For what is seen is temporary, but what is unseen is eternal (2 Corinthians 4:18).

The patient neither speaks nor comprehends the spoken word. Sometimes she babbles incoherently for hours on end. She is disoriented about person, place, and time. She does, however, respond to her own name. I have worked with her for the past six months, but she still shows no effort to assist in her own care. She must be completely fed, bathed, and clothed by others. She cannot control her bowels and bladder. Because she has no teeth, all her food must be pureed. Her clothing is usually soiled from incessant drooling.

She does not walk. Her sleep pattern is erratic. Often she wakes in the middle of the night and her screaming wakes others. Most of the time she is friendly and happy, but several times a day she gets quite agitated without apparent cause. Then she waits until someone comes to comfort her.

I asked other doctors and nurses how they would feel about taking care of such a patient. They used words like "hopeless," "frustrated," "depressed," and "annoyed." When I said that I enjoyed it and thought they would, too, they looked at me in disbelief. Then I passed around a picture of the "patient", my six-month-old daughter.

Why is it so much more difficult to care for a 90-year-old than a six-month-old with identical symptoms? A helpless baby may weigh 15 pounds and a helpless adult 150; but the answer goes deeper than this. The infant represents new life, hope, and almost infinite potential. The aged patient represents the end of life with little chance for change and growth because death is near. But wait! What is death? Is it not perhaps the greatest potential of all for change and growth? In Christ, death represents the end of the old, a new beginning: new life, hope, and infinite potential.

We need to see things from God's perspective. Those who are approaching the end of this life in the helplessness of old age need and deserve the same care and attention as those who are beginning their lives in the helplessness of infancy. I like the motto that Life Care Centers have adopted: "The sun setting is no less beautiful than the sun rising."

Originally shared at a nursing home training workshop. Author unknown. Adapted by Bill Goodrich for God Cares News

One of the greatest challenges for nursing-home volunteers is reaching out to residents who have dementia. Dementia is the loss of intellectual functions (thinking, remembering, and reasoning), of sufficient severity to interfere with an individual's daily functioning. Dementia is not a disease in itself, but rather a set of symptoms. Dementia may accompany certain diseases or conditions. Symptoms of dementia may also include changes in personality, mood, and behavior.

We tend to think that when people have dementia, they completely lose touch with all forms of reality. As a result, we may shy away from visiting or trying to minister to residents with this disorder. It is important to realize that the causes and rate of progression of dementia vary from one type of dementia to another. Memory loss usually associated with dementia can often be very gradual, and long-term memory retained for many years.

According to the Alzheimer's Association, some of the well-known diseases that may produce symptoms of dementia include: Alzheimer's Disease, Multi-Infarct Dementia, Parkinson's Disease, Huntington's Disease, Pick's Disease, Creutzfeldt-Jakob Disease, Amyotrophic Lateral Sclerosis (Lou Gehrig's Disease), and Multiple Sclerosis. Other conditions which can cause or mimic dementia include hydrocephalus, depression, thyroid disorders, nutritional deficiencies, infections (for example meningitis, syphilis, AIDS), alcoholism, brain tumors, head injuries, and drug reactions. Some of these conditions may be treatable or reversible.

All persons suspected of having dementia should receive a diagnostic examination. The examination can help determine the cause of the dementia and possible treatment; early diagnosis also helps families begin appropriate planning for future needs. Only those who have been close to a person who has suffered from a chronic dementia can really understand the devastation it can have on the family. Alzheimer's disease, for example, is often referred to as "the longest goodbye," as it saps the life and character of the person before the person actually physically dies.

Below we have described a few of the most common dementias you may find in the nursing home. A little working knowledge of these various conditions can help alleviate any concerns of visiting and of ministry.

Alzheimer's disease (AD)

Alzheimer's disease is a progressive, degenerative disease that attacks various structures in the brain and results in impaired memory and thought processes; as a result, behavior and personality are also affected. Approximately 4 million American adults suffer from Alzheimer's today. The Alzheimer's Association estimates that 14 million Americans will have Alzheimer's disease by the year 2050 if no prevention or cure is found. Approximately one out of every 10 persons over age 65, and nearly half of those over age 85 have Alzheimer's disease. Alzheimer's disease costs society more than $100 billion per year in health care and related costs. (See www.alz.org for more information).

AD usually has a gradual onset. Problems remembering recent events and difficulty performing familiar tasks are early symptoms. The person with Alzheimer's may also experience confusion, personality change, behavior change, and impaired judgment. Difficulty finding words, finishing thoughts or following directions are common. How quickly these changes occur will vary from person to person, but the disease eventually leaves its victims totally unable to care for themselves.

An absolute diagnosis can be made only through autopsy with a microscopic examination of brain tissue. Brains of people who have had Alzheimer's exhibit the characteristic signs of senile plaques and neurofibrillary tangles in those areas of the brain responsible for memory and intellectual functions. Alzheimer's patients have also been found to lack acetylcholine, a chemical which is involved in the processing of memory, especially short-term memory.

> **THE ALZHEIMER'S ASSOCIATION**
>
> Alzheimer's Association has a network of more than 200 chapters nationwide, providing programs and services within their communities that assist persons with Alzheimer's disease, their families and caregivers. These programs and services include support groups, telephone help lines, educational seminars, and a variety of publications on the disease, on current research, caregiving approaches and more.

Multi-infarct dementia (MID)

Multi-infarct dementia, or vascular dementia, is mental deterioration caused by multiple strokes (infarcts) in the brain. This is the second most common form of dementia. The onset of MID may be relatively sudden as many strokes can occur before symptoms appear. These strokes may damage areas of the brain responsible for a specific function, such as the ability to calculate, and there may be more generalized symptoms, such as disorientation, confusion, and behavioral changes. MID symptoms may appear similar to Alzheimer's disease. MID and Alzheimer's disease co-exist in 15-25 percent of dementia patients.

Brain scan techniques like computerized axial tomography (CAT scans) and magnetic resonance imaging (MRIs) are used to identify strokes in the brain. MID progresses in downhill steps with plateaus or periods of stability, with possibly some slight improvement between strokes.

High blood pressure, vascular disease, diabetes or previous strokes have been identified as risk factors for MID. It is not reversible or curable, but treatment of underlying conditions (e.g., antihypertensive medication) may halt progression and prevent further strokes.

Parkinson's disease (PD)

Individuals with Parkinson's disease lack a substance called dopamine. Dopamine helps control muscle activity by the nervous system. Tremors, stiffness and slowness of movement are characteristic features of Parkinson's disease. Speech may also be slow. Movement may be difficult to initiate. Late in the course of the disease some people with Parkinson's, though not all, may develop dementia. Parkinson drugs can improve motor symptoms but do not improve the mental changes that occur.

Depression

Depression is a mood disorder marked by sadness, inactivity, difficulty in thinking and concentration, feelings of hopelessness, and, if severe, suicidal tendencies. Many severely depressed patients will have poor concentration and attention. When dementia and depression are present together, intellectual deterioration may be exaggerated. Depression, whether present alone or in combination with dementia, can often be effectively treated with medications like antidepressants. This is often neglected in people with dementia, but the possibility of depression should be assessed. There are, of course, many other interventions that can be helpful to help alleviate depression, including the presence of a caring friend.

PERSPECTIVES ON DEMENTIA

The apostle Paul said,

> ***"Be transformed by the renewing of your mind. Then you will be able to test and approve what God's will is...." (Romans 12:2).***

But what if the mind can no longer be renewed? Can people still be spiritually transformed with the ability to test and approve God's will? We believe the answer is yes.

The spiritual needs of persons who have cognitive or mental impairment are the same as the spiritual needs of those who are more fully cognitively functional. If the cognitive or intellectual part of a person is deemed *exclusively important,* spiritual needs can easily be ignored for those who are cognitively impaired.

The method of meeting these spiritual needs may differ, however, even though the needs themselves are the same. When these needs are creatively met, this can be a great source of comfort, joy and hope for the person with a dementia as well as their family members.

WHY ARE WE UNCOMFORTABLE?

There is often a temptation to shy away from people who have dementia for the following reasons:

- We feel awkward and uncomfortable with behavior and personality change associated with dementia.
- We do not know what say to someone who may not be able to respond verbally.
- We assume a person with dementia cannot understand any of our words.
- We don't see the point of listening to a person who is cognitively impaired when we don't understand what they are saying.
- We are afraid the disease associated with dementia symptoms might be contagious.
- We are afraid of facing our own frailty.
- We are afraid that we won't understand what the person is saying, and therefore will not be able to respond without embarrassing him or ourselves.

In spite of our own fears and the physical and mental frailties of the other person, there is much evidence that we are able to provide quality spiritual care through the love and Word of God.

EFFECTIVE MINISTRY IS POSSIBLE

There are different kinds of dementia, there are also different levels of severity. When we make assumptions or judgments about people's cognitive ability before we take the time to get to know them, we can very easily neglect the opportunity to minister life, hope, joy and peace. We must come alongside each individual and share with him according to the person's unique needs and ability.

For instance, one might make the false assumption that a person who has had a stroke that has affected his ability to speak has some form of dementia based on outward expressions and appearance. But, contrary to the expressions and appearances, the person may have total ability to understand, though not the ability to express his thoughts into understandable words or expressions. It might seem as if you are trying to communicate with a person who can speak only a foreign language. The person's inability to help you to understand does not mean the person doesn't know what is going on around him.

Similarly, some people affected with dementia are not able to speak any words at all, but may have non-verbal ways to communicate. There are even many cases of people who have come out of a coma and testified that they heard all that was going on around them, even when doctors would be making medical decisions with the family in the same room, assuming the patient was brain-dead.

Although a person may seem not to understand what is going on around him, we must respect and treat him the way we would want to be treated and trust that he can both hear and understand us. Perhaps, only in heaven, will he be able to thank us.

What we have found with many people who are challenged by a dementia, particularly in the early stages, is that they realize they have a communication problem and are often very frustrated because they want to share verbally as they did before their illness. It is a great blessing to them when someone takes the time to get close enough and is creative enough to truly observe and listen. If we can somehow be patient and learn their unspoken or sometimes fractured language, we can give them an opportunity to express themselves. Our experience is that we rarely completely understand all they have to say. We can, however, often discover and appropriately respond to the general meaning of partial words, phrases and body language. The following impressions shared by a caregiver illustrate these points:

> *"More and more I am coming to understand that the needs of our dementia population are the same as the needs of our youngest population. They need to be spoken to gently, with real love and affection. They need to be caressed and touched...their hands held and their cheeks kissed tenderly. They need to joke, laugh and have fun, which is not always easy to do. They like to have us laugh at their humor, even if we cannot understand the words, only the inflection...to be the life of the party, even though the party is a simple gathering in an Alzheimer's home. They need us to be honest with them. They can spot a phony in a minute. They need to be able to succeed at what they do, even if all they are able to do is walk around the room, walk to their chair, or eat their dinner. Success is as important to them as it is to us. Bottom line—they need us, as we need them...their... innocence and love, enrich us beyond belief."*
> *Victoria McCarty, Care Tender, August 2000*

Some residents do and say things that do not seem sensible to us. One might say he wants to go home to his mother and may even attempt to leave the nursing home, when in reality, his mother died several years ago. Some dementia victims go into what appears to be a dream-like state, in the sense that things that are not real become real to them. This can be frustrating for the person who is trying to make sense out of their reality. Their reality will normally produce emotions and behaviors that are sometimes challenging for the visitor as well as the nursing home staff. It is important for us to walk a while in our friends' reality, understand as much as possible and validate their emotions and concerns. In doing so, we establish trust. We do not reinforce false beliefs and perceptions, but we can affirm our understanding of their reality. Depending on the degree of dementia, we may, at times, be able to gradually redirect them into reality. The following is an example:

> *A woman in a nursing home was struggling because she believed that she needed to catch the bus to get home. She was upset because members of the nursing staff were telling her that she could not leave, and they were trying to get her to sit down and watch the television. They were very ineffective in their efforts to divert her attention and she was starting to get aggressive with them.*
>
> *I (Bill) knew that she could not leave and that there was no bus to catch, but I decided to spend some time with her to listen to her concerns. What she said was that she was out of money and needed to leave because she could not afford the room for the night. After applying some principles of validation, in just a few minutes, I gained her trust and was able to assure her that not only was the room paid for that night but also her dinner and breakfast were covered. I also assured her that Jesus loved her and that He would help her when things get frustrating. She accepted my words and went away in peace, singing a song.*
>
> *I have had to do the same kind of thing for her over and over and over again in the past year. Some may think that this is frustrating, but I see the fruit of God in it because she is comforted by the love of God. Each time I talk with her, I tell*

her something about Jesus. When she is reminded that He loves her and will help her, she seems to find much comfort. Although I have all of my cognitive functions (at least I think I do), I too find much comfort in being reminded that Jesus loves me and that He is near in the midst of my times of confusion.

Some may grow weary from having to go through this same process over and over, or to hear the same stories over and over. But we must remember that **"It is more blessed to give than it is to receive"** *(Acts 20:35).*

VALIDATION MINISTRY

It is easy to be at a loss for words and a proper response while visiting someone who has dementia. The technique of validation can assist you. Validation ministry is an attitude and also a method that works to earn the trust of confused people. We address their concerns with compassion and empathy and, when appropriate, we redirect their attention toward reality.

Validation is, essentially, treating people the way we would want to be treated if we were confused. With validation, we do not confront people with conflicting information; instead we try to enter into their reality by **active listening**.

We actively listen by:

- Listening with our hearts, eyes and our expressions. (See Chapter 5 for more information on listening with our heart and responding in love.)

- Prayerfully discerning what the Lord wants to do. We know that the Lord understands the confused person. We need to ask Him to give us insight and to touch our friend through us.

It is also very possible that our friend may be troubled with the reality of unresolved conflicts in his life, yet lacks the ability to communicate these concerns appropriately. As with most of us who struggle with the challenges of life, we do not trust just anybody with our deep concerns. Only with a trusted friend who compassionately understands will we risk sharing and seeking help. In our role as visitor (not professional counselor) some of these conflicts may surface. Our role is to listen and **validate** feelings and, when appropriate, share words of hope.

> *Thou wilt keep him in perfect peace, whose mind is stayed on thee: because he trusteth in thee.*
> *Isaiah 26:3* KJV

We validate by:

- Expressing sincere words of empathy.
- Sometimes repeating in our own words what we understand our friend is saying can help him to realize that we understand his situation. Remember, we do not know how another person feels, but we can often come to some understanding of his concerns if we truly listen and reflect.
- Walking awhile in his reality and helping him to realize that you care about him.
- Not making light of his troubles, no matter how insignificant they may seem or how inappropriately they may be expressed. Painful feelings that are expressed, and validated by a friend, will often diminish in time. When ignored, they will oftentimes gain strength.

Active listening through validation can help our friend realize that we care and understand his concerns and that we are interested in his welfare. This may earn us the trust needed to **redirect** him to a more realistic perspective of his concerns.

We can redirect our friend:

- When there is a connection of hearts.
- Through the use of calm and assuring words or focusing on items of interest.
- With patience. Don't be in a hurry.
- Prayerfully. As we pray, the Holy Spirit can guide us to reassuring Scriptures to read and/or songs to share that may result in peace and hope.
- In the role of a helper, not a counselor. We are friends who care and know the Lord Jesus. As we listen and validate and share from Scripture and from our own lives, we are ultimately pointing our friend to the only reality that promises true peace, JESUS. **(John 14:27, John 16:33)**
- With realities such as the following:
    - Jesus loves you
    - Jesus cares about your concerns
    - Jesus will help if we ask Him
    - Jesus will help you because He promised to
    - Jesus said, "Trust in Me."

A friend may be trying to find his mother when it is quite obvious that she no longer lives. The fact that this mother is not living anymore is not necessarily a reality that needs to be addressed or corrected. You can ask questions about his mother to see if there are any concerns about which to pray. It is appropriate to say, "Tell me more about your mother." The person may then begin to reminisce about past experiences, and you can gain more insight into their relationships and possible needs.

Validation ministry is an art that we should learn and practice as we reach out to our friends in the nursing home. These principles may also apply to our neighbors or loved ones who are confused and deeply troubled by life's challenges, or who may not have a personal relationship with Jesus. The more we lovingly validate our friend's concerns, the more we will see God's Word have a life-changing effect.

> Naomi Feil ACSW, has been developing the practice of validation since 1963. Many of her principles have been adapted and used for this section.

COMMUNICATION

In all Christian outreach, we are ultimately seeking to communicate God's Word in such a way that those who hear might turn to Jesus, or walk closer to Him. Communication is the way we share ourselves with others. There are various ways to communicate. The most recognized way is through speech and hearing. However, body language, tone of voice, touch, and attitude are also ways we communicate. A person can say all the right words, but if you sense that he is looking down on you, or patronizing you, you may not want to receive his words. Some studies estimate that only 20% of our communication is verbal. The other 80% of communication consists of things like voice tone, body language, and attitude. Jesus communicated the full extent of His love by an action, i.e. washing His disciples' feet *(John 13:1-5)*. St. Francis of Assisi said; "Wherever you go, preach the gospel, and whenever necessary, use words." Paul wrote,

> **"If I speak with tongues of men and of angels and do not have love, I am only a resounding gong or a clanging cymbal" (1Corinthians 13:1).**

> Remember that your genuine interest and caring make their impact on the heart regardless of the person's state of mind.
> Tom and Kaye DePinto, Nursing Home Ministry

Tips for more effective communication

As messengers of the Gospel, we must learn to impart or transmit what God speaks to us in order to edify the body of Christ. Even though some residents will not be able to respond with appropriate words, they are often able to understand much of what we say. When we communicate, we are not only speaking words, we are also transmitting our spirit. Our love, patience, and even anger can often impact people more than our words. The following are some tips for more effective communication with people with dementia:

1. Body language is very important. Try to position yourself at eye level with a cheerful countenance. If the resident is upset or confused, try to respond to the emotion that you see. Let him see in your eyes that you really care, but do not treat the resident as a child.

2. Do not assume a resident has certain disabilities such as impaired hearing or loss of comprehension skills. Approach the resident as if there are no disabilities and make adjustments as you see the need.

3. Once your friend is able to trust you, he may be comforted by a gentle hug, touch on the shoulder or a hand to hold.

4. If your friend begins to talk about things unrelated to the conversation, don't abruptly correct him. It is often quite effective to walk for a while in his reality, rather than hastily lead him into your reality. Remember that validation ministry may work well for some residents, but not with others, especially those with severe dementia. This is a result of the disease process and damaged brain cells.

5. Allow your friend time to comprehend what you are saying. If need be, rephrase your sentence or question to help him understand. Do not allow him to struggle too long for the right words. Sometimes it is good to help him with a word or phrase or politely excuse him from having

to answer your questions. In the early stages of the disability, people with dementia are usually very sensitive, so avoid making them feel inadequate or overly self-conscious.

6. Try to reduce background noises, which can distract or cause confusion. Visiting one-to-one may also reduce confusion. You may need to turn off a television or turn down a radio. Be sure to ask permission. You may also need to relocate a resident if other residents are noisy and distracting. Residents often enjoy being wheeled outside. Generally, the nursing home has a court-yard or patio. (Remember, however, that people with dementia may wander away and put themselves in danger. NEVER leave a resident with dementia unattended, if you have taken him outside). Make sure they bring a sweater or blanket or are otherwise appropriately dressed for the weather conditions.

7. Be sensitive while holding conversations with others in your friend's presence as if he were not there. Difficulties in understanding all that is being said could make him think that you are talking about him. Try to include him in the conversation.

8. It is usually good to read Scripture and pray for your friend, but this does not have to happen at every visit. It is best to read the Scripture that pertains to the need at the moment and let the Lord reveal His truth. It is helpful to use a Bible translation that is easily understood such as NIV (New International Version) or NLT (New Living Translation) or NKJV (New King James Version), unless you discern that your friend prefers the traditional KJV. Residents with dementia may have memorized Scripture from the KJV and might still be able to recite it.

9. Never underestimate the power of the spoken Word of God. Speak the Word with gentleness and in faith, believing that the Word of God can cut through earthly limitations, including those of dementia.

10. Many good messages and prayers are in the old hymns. Many residents who cannot talk can still sing and may remember all the verses of a hymn. The Lord's Prayer and the 23rd Psalm are also usually remembered Scripture passages. A resident may be able to recite these with you or even alone if you initiate this with him. Both hymns and Scriptures can be of great comfort as together you focus on the familiar.
11. The Lord knows the residents and their needs. Our primary role is to pray and take steps of faith as the Holy Spirit guides us to bless them. Above all:

Treat others the way you would like to be treated (James 2:8).

The following example illustrates a number of the foregoing points:

Once, I (Tom), was sitting with a woman who was in a wheelchair and was very much in her own reality. Having tried to enter her reality unsuccessfully, the thought occurred to me to begin reciting the 23rd Psalm. I did so, slowly and quietly...and in English. About the second verse, I was joined by this woman reciting the 23rd Psalm in German. After we finished, with me lowering my voice to allow her German recitation to continue unimpeded, we had a wonderful conversation (in English) about her life in Germany, her husband's ice cream store, including the favorite flavors, her Church and her love for Jesus. Shortly after sharing this very sweet time of coherence, she lapsed again into her own reality. I held her hand for a while, said a brief prayer, and left with a wonderful sense of peace and gratitude.

THE MINISTRY OF THE WORD OF GOD

It can appear that sharing the gospel with people who have dementia is rather fruitless, because they do not appear to have the ability to comprehend the Word of God. We need to remember that even people who have all their mental functions intact cannot grasp the great things of God unless the Lord chooses to reveal them. This is true today and has been true throughout history. Once Jesus prayed:

> *"I praise you, Father, Lord of heaven and earth, because you have hidden these things from the wise and learned, and revealed them to little children. Yes, Father, for this was your good pleasure. All things have been committed to me by my Father. No one knows the Son except the Father, and no one knows the Father except the Son and those to whom the Son chooses to reveal him" (Matthew 11:25-27).*

This Scripture passage holds the key to ministering effectively to people who have dementia. If Jesus chooses to reveal Himself and the Father, He is able to do so in spite of our limitations. One wonderful part of this blessing is that the Lord chooses to use us to accomplish His great work.

Helping people with dementia connect with Jesus is not done by any special three-or four-step evangelistic program, but by faith, love, and the leading and guiding of the Holy Spirit. We must never underestimate the power of God's Word to break through dementia and have a positive and life-changing effect.

Two Scriptures that remind us of this:

> *The words I have spoken to you are spirit and they are life (John 6:63).*

For the Word of God is living and active. Sharper than any double-edged sword, it penetrates even to dividing soul and spirit, joints and marrow... (Hebrews 4:12).

A BIBLE STUDY THAT BREAKS THROUGH

Below is a testimony of how the Lord has been using a few women to impart life to their friends living in an Alzheimer's unit.

We minister in an Alzheimer's unit at a nursing home nearby. All of the people in the unit have some form of dementia which varies from being totally unresponsive to very aware of what is going on around them.

We've been going there once a week for seven years. We share a devotional in the unit for 45 minutes or so, and we also visit people on the way in and on the way out. We are there about an hour and a half. Our service in the unit is just before dinner 4:00 to 4:45 so the staff usually have the residents all gathered in the dining room by the time we get there. The staff is very helpful. They tell us they really appreciate our visits.

There are five ladies on our team. Usually three or four are there for each service, but sometimes just one or two. God always blesses our time there, no matter how many team members we have. Sometimes we take our children or grandchildren and that's always an added blessing. Some of the people who are usually still and unresponsive respond to the children. The devotional format is flexible, but generally goes as follows:

We begin with prayer, then while handing out the paper that has the Scripture reading for the day, we sing, "Jesus Loves Me." Then we read the message and ask the folks to follow along. Some do, some just listen, some sleep.

Presently, we are sharing a Psalm each week. We give a very short devotional related to the Word and end with a prayer that is written on the bottom of the page. I always tell them that God blesses us because we come together in the name of Jesus.

For the worship music, we have a tape with ten songs (we sing the same songs every week). Some of the songs are, "O How I Love Jesus," "To Be Like Jesus," "I Have Decided to Follow Jesus," "Lift Jesus Higher," and "He is Lord." We end by singing, "God Bless America". I tell the people that this song, "God Bless America," is our prayer for everyone who lives in this country and that they are doing something very important when they sing it.

After we sing the last song, we go around to each person there and say, "God bless you" and talk with those who want to. It is a very blessed fellowship. The people receive us with much kindness and appreciation. We then visit other residents throughout the unit and the rest of the nursing home. We pray with them individually if they are upset or ill, or when they are dying. We also pray with the families when they ask us to.

Many residents thank us for bringing the Word and the music. Many who cannot even say their own names will listen very closely when I talk to them and at the end will say, "God bless you" or "Thank you for coming" to me. It's very important to take the time to wait for them to respond. We always take their hand and look in their eyes so they know that we care about each one. We go to every person in the room. We know their names because the nurses tell us or it's on the door of their room.

> In this kind of ministry, we must always remember what Jesus said in **Matthew 25:40, "Whatever you did for one of the least of these brothers of mine you did for me."** They are no less than other people because they are in the nursing home. They are just less fortunate because they are unable to take care of themselves and be independent any longer. Therefore, we must go to them.
>
> It is such a blessing and privilege to carry the Gospel to our brothers and sisters and those who may not know Jesus yet. As we are faithful to love as Jesus taught us, the people who live in these homes and those who work there will come to know Him. Jesus said, **"If I be lifted up.. I will draw all men to myself"** (John 12:32).
>
> I love to go there even when I'm very busy, or tired, or under a lot of stress. God always blesses all of us. We see the suffering of our brothers and sisters and their declining health, but we also see the power of God to lift all of our spirits as we share His love with each other.
>
> God has taught us in **Matthew 7:12, "In everything do to others what you would have them do to you."** If I were there in the nursing home, I would want someone to come and share the Word of God with me, and sing with me, and tell me "God loves you," and "Jesus loves you, and so do I." That's why I go while I still can.
>
> Mary Ann Goodrich

Researchers have discovered that people with Alzheimer's will lose their long-term memory as the disease progresses. Long-term memory may include things for people like their own name, their parents' names, their ABC's and perhaps some basic spelling or arithmetic. These are normally learned before the age of seven. Many people in the later stages of AD cannot remember any of these. They often will not be able to remember that they even have a spouse or children. Yet many of these same people can sing a hymn or even quote a Bible verse like **John 3:16, Psalm 23** or the Lord's Prayer. There is something special about the Word and the Spirit of God that is not well understood by modern science. Perhaps many of these spiritual things are treasured in the heart and when the mind is broken, the heart still expresses itself.

*Once after a Bible study in an Alzheimer's unit, a woman who was severely demented was staring at the Scripture verses that were written on paper. After several minutes of intense staring, she looked up and announced, "This is an excellent philosophy. Everyone should read this!" That was an incredible statement from someone living in an Alzheimer's unit, especially when men and woman with high IQ's have read God's Word and rejected it. Indeed God reveals His truth to little children and hides it from the learned **(Luke 10:21).** Mary Ann Goodrich*

Brothers, think of what you were when you were called. Not many of you were wise by human standards; not many were influential; not many were of noble birth. But God chose the foolish things of the world to shame the wise; God chose the weak things of the world to shame the strong. He chose the lowly things of this world and the despised things--and the things that are not--to nullify the things that are, so that no one may boast before him.

1Corinthians 1:26-29

WE MINISTER BY FAITH AND NOT BY SIGHT

Please take the time to read **John 11:1-44** so that the following principles may have deeper significance for you. The following points are highlights from this passage:

- Jesus received a message that His close friend Lazarus was very sick.
- Mary and Martha requested that Jesus come to see Lazarus.
- Jesus promised that Lazarus' sickness would not end in death.
- When Jesus finally arrived, He found that Lazarus was already dead for four days.
- Martha went out to meet Jesus and while expressing her grief, Jesus assured her that Lazarus would rise.

"Jesus said to her, 'Your brother will rise again.' Martha answered, 'I know he will rise again in the resurrection at the last day.' Jesus said to her, 'I am the resurrection and the life. He who believes in me will live, even though he dies; and whoever lives and believes in me will never die. Do you believe this?'" (John 11: 23-26).

- Later, Mary went out to meet Jesus and He followed her to Lazarus's tomb.
- Jesus was moved with grief and tears as He approached the tomb.

"Jesus, once more deeply moved, came to the tomb. It was a cave with a stone laid across the entrance. 'Take away the stone,' he said. 'But, Lord,' said Martha, the sister of the dead man, 'by this time there is a bad odor, for he has been there four days.' Then Jesus said, 'Did I not tell

you that if you believed, you would see the glory of God?' So they took away the stone. Then Jesus looked up and said, 'Father, I thank you that you have heard me. I knew that you always hear me, but I said this for the benefit of the people standing here, that they may believe that you sent me.' When he had said this, Jesus called in a loud voice, 'Lazarus, come out!' The dead man came out, his hands and feet wrapped with strips of linen, and a cloth around his face. Jesus said to them, 'Take off the grave clothes and let him go.'" *(John 11:38-44).*

The review of this Bible story is important because it reveals the same principles we must apply when ministering to our friends who have dementia. There are at least four things that Jesus did before Lazarus rose from the dead:

1. He obeyed the Father.
2. Although He understood the reality of the death of Lazarus, He acted in faith.
3. He involved other people. By faith they obeyed and did what they could do.
4. Jesus spoke His Words of life.

As a result of what Jesus said and did, death had no power. The Word of God was more powerful. By the Word of the Lord, this man lived.

The Word of God is not just an intellectual expression. The Word of God is spirit and it penetrates beyond the body and the mind into the soul of men. Indeed, people receive Jesus into their hearts, not just their minds. It is our conviction then, that when the Word of the Lord is shared in a spirit of love, it is as if we are feeding a person with dementia "intravenously"— straight to the heart! By faith, we trust and have often seen convincing evidence that God's Word breaks through.

When Jesus spoke to Lazarus, did Lazarus hear Jesus with his physical ears or did Jesus' Word enter his mind so that he could conclude that it was time to wake up? Certainly NOT! The Word of Jesus was so powerful that it bypassed or cut through the physical, moving into the place of the spirit, commanding even death to step aside. Jesus' Word is so powerful that if He did not specify Lazarus, and would have just commanded, *"Come out,"* everyone else in the graves nearby would have risen as well. Jesus said, *"Did I not tell you that if you believed, you would see the glory of God?" John 11:40.* By the Word of God, Lazarus lived.

Jesus gave us His Word to speak and bring life, but we must first be willing to remove the stone of science and technology that implies there is no hope. We must be careful not to lean totally on the understanding of man's discoveries or lack of discoveries. We must lean on the Lord of life (**Proverbs 3:5-6**).

If we want to see the glory of God, we must act in faith. By faith we do what is possible (speaking the Word of God, even when it seems hopeless), and the Lord does what is impossible (breathes life into the soul). God is faithful. We just need to do what He says and we will see His glory.

This principle is also clearly expressed in **Mark 5:21-24, 35-42** and **Ezekiel 37:1-14**.

It does not, therefore, depend on man's desire or effort, but on God's mercy (Romans 9:15).

TAPPING INTO DIVINE POWER

When we are abiding in Christ, we have access to divine power. This is the power needed to minister beyond the limitations of dementia. There are at least seven ways this divine power is available to us:

1) Through the Name of Jesus:

The Father has sent His son Jesus. He has given Jesus authority to protect and bless, and it is through the name of Jesus that life, hope, and peace are imparted.

> *Therefore God exalted him to the highest place and gave him the name that is above every name, that at the name of Jesus every knee should bow, in heaven and on earth and under the earth, and every tongue confess that Jesus Christ is Lord, to the glory of God the Father (Philippians 2:9-11).*

2) Through the Word of the Lord:

The Word of the Lord is not just an intellectual expression. Rather, the Word of the Lord is a spiritual word that brings forth life.

> *The Spirit gives life; the flesh counts for nothing. The words I have spoken to you are spirit and they are life (John 6:63).*

3) Through Prayer:

Prayer is not just a ritual that gives a person a sense of connection with God. Prayer is communication with our Father in heaven. The Lord hears the cry of His children.

> *They were helped in fighting them, and God handed the Hagrites and all their allies over to them, because they cried out to him during the battle. He answered their prayers, because they trusted in him (1 Chronicles 5:20).*

4) Through Faith:

Everything we do in Christ starts out with a step of faith. After a few steps of faith, understanding and wisdom follow. It is through faith that we will see the power of God's Word.

> *Now faith is being sure of what we hope for and certain of what we do not see (Hebrews 11:1).*

5) Through Hope:

Hope has power that most do not realize. Hope enables us to go beyond normal limitations. But our hope must be in the Lord who gave us His principles and promises.

> *But those who hope in the LORD will renew their strength. They will soar on wings like eagles; they will run and not grow weary, they will walk and not be faint (Isaiah 40:31).*

6) Through Love:

God Himself is love. Those who live in love, live in God. When we are acting in God's love, God is moving through us **(1 John 4:7-21)**.

> *Love never fails... And now these three remain: faith, hope and love. But the greatest of these is love (1 Corinthians 13:8,13).*

7) Through the Holy Spirit:

Our Father speaks to us and guides us to join Him in what He is doing through His Spirit. The Holy Spirit will guide, counsel, and enable us to minister effectively the love and Word of God.

> *This is the Word of the LORD to Zerubbabel: "Not by might nor by power, but by my Spirit," says the LORD Almighty (Zechariah 4:6).*

Jesus relied on the same resources when He ministered on earth. These resources are heavenly treasures that our Father imparts to us as we abide in the True Vine **(John 15:1)**. As we realize our inability to minister to others in our own power, we cry out for the Lord's help and seek His Word and grace. This is when His treasures are imparted to us. We do what is possible out of love and obedience and God does what is impossible according to His divine will.

If by the Spirit of love, we prayerfully go in faith and in the name of our Lord Jesus Christ, to share His Word, and to lift up His name with our friends, having deep hope that they will draw near to our Father, the rest is up to the LORD.

CONCERNING THEIR SALVATION

*Over the years, I (Bill) have ministered to hundreds of nursing home residents who have had some form of dementia. Sam was one such soul who was diagnosed with Alzheimer's disease. When I entered the nursing home to visit a friend's mother, Sam greeted me by saying, "I want to go home." Since I did not know him and this was my first time to go to the nursing home, and my friend was trying to lead me to his mother's room, I tried to avoid Sam. He persisted, and compassion would not let me just go by. I began to look for a way to encourage Sam by redirecting his focus to a more manageable subject. I was very ineffective because he kept returning to the subject of wanting to go home. The way that he said, "I want to go home," reminded me of what Jesus said in **John 14**. I asked Sam, "Are you ready to go home?" He looked at me a little puzzled and I continued, "Someone wants to come to take you home, but you need to get yourself ready." Then I asked, "Do you want me to tell you how to get ready? The one who wants to take you home is Jesus, and the way to get ready is to ask Him to help you get ready. Would you like to do that?" After a little more conversation, we bowed our hearts in prayer. I prayed for Sam, then led him in a prayer to receive Jesus into his heart and prepare him for the time when Jesus will come to take him home. What a blessing it was for all of us! My friend who was inexperienced with this kind of ministry was amazed (so was I). I never* *did see Sam again, but I do trust I will meet him again with a sound mind and in the presence of our Lord.*

"In my Father's house are many rooms; if it were not so, I would have told you. I am going there to prepare a place for you. And if I go and prepare a place for you, I will come back and take you to be with me that you also may be where I am" (John 14:2-3).

For Sam, his salvation did not come because he understood Biblical principles and concepts. It came as a result of someone pointing him to Jesus on his level. Once he realized his need was greater then his ability, he asked Jesus for help, for *"Everyone who calls on the name of the Lord will be saved" (Romans 10:13).*

Jesus said that all men will know we are His disciples by our love **(John 13:35).** When we go to the nursing home in the name of Jesus, speaking the Word of God in Christian love, and a resident receives us, he in turn is receiving Jesus. Jesus said, *"He who receives you receives me, and he who receives me receives the one who sent me" Matthew 10:40.*

For most of us, the beginning of our personal relationship with the Lord started with our praying a humble prayer of repentance from our sin and then committing our lives by faith into Jesus' care. In this prayer, we repented of our sins and committed to follow Jesus. Millions have been introduced to Jesus in this way. However, we want to emphasize that although this kind of sinner's prayer is based on Biblical principles, **it is not specifically written in the Bible** that a person must say the sinner's prayer to be saved. What God did say is, *"To all who received Him and believed in Jesus' name, He gave them the right to become children of God" (John 1:12-13).*

Our Father in heaven is able to reveal Himself to anyone, regardless of mental limitations. *It (our salvation) does not, therefore, depend on man's desire or effort, but on God's mercy (Romans 9:16).* Therefore, when we come to a person who does not have the ability to respond by praying a particular form of the "Sinner's Prayer," we must be willing to trust our merciful Savior to judge the thoughts and intents of his heart and make a righteous and merciful judgment.

These are other important Scriptures to consider:

Jesus replied, "Blessed are you, Simon son of Jonah, for this was not revealed to you by man, but by my Father in heaven" (Matthew 16:17).

No eye has seen, no ear has heard, no mind has conceived what God has prepared for those who love him—but God has revealed it to us by his Spirit (1 Corinthians 2:9-10).

For there is no difference between Jew and Gentile-- the same Lord is Lord of all and richly blesses all who call on him (Romans 10:12).

And everyone who calls on the name of the Lord will be saved (Acts 2:21).

Applying the above principles is no guarantee that we will see the desired results. There are times we can only hope that our efforts are making a difference. Our hope is that our friends, who were not able to respond verbally to the Lord as we knelt at their bedside to pray for them, will one day respond with all of their being to the Lord in heaven. The thought of that wonderful future can make our joy complete!

> *One lady (Millie) hardly says anything. I (Bill) go into her room and speak softly into her ear and say, "Millie, we're going to have a church service. Come with me and hear about Jesus." When she hears His name, she smiles and says, "Jesus." Yes, that's almost all I can remember Millie saying in three years. She does not sing or quote Bible verses. She just smiles and says "Jesus" when I speak His name to her. She's beautiful!*

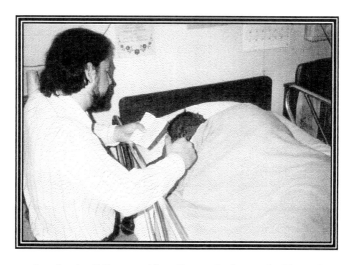

Against all hope, Abraham, in hope believed..
(Romans 4:18).

CHAPTER 9

RECRUITING HELP AND RETAINING IT

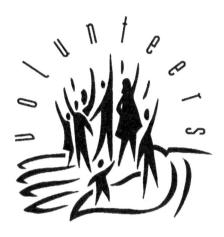

Our church has several care teams. We come together once a month to make crafts for the residents, fellowship, and pray for one another and the ministry. We are family! Several of us have been with the ministry for over ten years."
                                        Chris Callahan

One time a resident wrote a short letter for me (Bill) to read to my church as I was presenting the need for more team members. In a very direct way, she urged them to take some time to come to the nursing home, fellowship with them, and see the ministry with their own eyes. A letter like this can be a good seed for recruiting new help. Paul, in Acts 16:6-10, had a vision in the night of a Macedonian standing and pleading with him saying, "Come on over to Macedonia and help us." When Paul had seen the vision, he and Silas immediately set out for Macedonia, concluding

that God had called them to preach the gospel. A similar cry can be heard in nursing homes every week. The letter from this resident was a good example of a Macedonian cry.

As we settle in and adjust to the environment of the nursing home, it doesn't take very long before we begin to understand the heart of Jesus and to realize the meaning of His Words to His disciples:

When Jesus saw the crowds, he had compassion on them, because they were harassed and helpless, like sheep without a shepherd. Then he said to his disciples, "The harvest is plentiful but the workers are few. Ask the Lord of the harvest, therefore, to send out workers into his harvest field." (Matthew 9:36-38).

The most frequent prayer request we receive from individuals at our training workshops and through letters is related to the need for more workers to help on ministry care teams. For most of us, recruiting volunteers usually rates from not easy to very frustrating. Throughout the years we have learned that there is little we can do to make recruiting easy. However, there are ways to make it more successful.

Being well organized and adopting the following guidelines will greatly assist your recruiting efforts. You will need to undergird your efforts with prayer and add a dose of creativity as you decide what is best for your needs and circumstances. Remember, the Lord of the Harvest is with you as you abide in the True Vine.

An estimated 35% of people ministering in nursing homes started as a result of a personal invitation from an experienced volunteer who needed help.

Recruiting volunteers is often done one person at a time.

Recruiting church members for the care team can be done simply by approaching individuals in your church and inviting them to join you. Another way is by presenting the ministry to the church and giving members an opportunity to sign up. This latter approach is recommended, as it will also give the ministry good visibility.

RECRUITING YOUR PASTOR

If you are going to establish or develop a care team within your church, you must have your pastor's support. The absence of pastoral support has been the primary reason many nursing-home ministries have not flourished.

According to **Ephesians 4:11-12**, pastors are responsible to facilitate, but not necessarily operate, ministries of helps like nursing-home outreach. In larger churches, there are usually Assistant Pastors or Deacons who support the Senior Pastor by overseeing outreach ministries. Whatever the case, when you approach the appropriate people about establishing a care team, it is important they understand that you and the team are planning to do the work, and what you need from them is their blessing and support. Pastors and other church leaders will need to have confidence that you will conduct yourself in a manner worthy of the gospel of Christ as you represent the church in the nursing home **(Philippians 1:27)**.

Presentation

When you present the ministry to your pastor, the pastor is likely going to ask:

1. What is the need?
2. What can be done to meet the need?

3. How do you want to meet the need?
4. Is meeting this need something the Lord wants our church to do?
5. How does this opportunity fit in with our church's vision?

You should have a fair understanding of these five questions and have the ability to respond to each of them in a short yet concise manner. Possible responses could be:

1. There is a nursing home in our community that has about 100 residents. Many of these people are facing death and are experiencing hopelessness, loneliness, and fear. Approximately 25% of the residents there have no church affiliation.
2. Every nursing home resident needs a friend to share the love and Word of God with them and give them hope.
3. With just four to six people, we can start a care team that visits the nursing home on a regular basis to share a Bible study, conduct a worship service and visit one-to-one. Showing your pastor the description of a nursing-home-ministry care team in Chapter 6 may also help.
4. The Lord has commanded us to care for people in distress and He promises to bless us if we obey. The Lord said, *"Do to others as you would have them do for you." Luke 6:31.* Scripture passages like **Matthew 25:31-45 and James 1:27** also speak of our responsibility to help nursing home residents. Scripture also commands us to honor our father and our mother; many nursing home residents have no children to honor them; this then becomes the responsibility of others, including the local church.
5. A nursing home ministry is an opportunity to make a positive difference in our community.

Timing

Timing is another important issue. The worst possible time to present your vision is after the Sunday worship service when your pastor's responsibility is service to the church body. He will appreciate not being forced to consider other issues that might distract from a focus on the present needs of the congregation. Call the church during the week and make an appointment to see your pastor. Briefly mention the purpose of your visit, but save your presentation for the meeting. You might also include testimonies from your own or others' experiences and bring some literature on nursing home ministry.

Prayer is also vitally important. The prayer of Nehemiah is an especially relevant one before you speak with your pastor or other church leaders:

> ***O Lord, let your ear be attentive to the prayer of this your servant and to the prayer of your servants who delight in revering your name. Give your servant success today by granting him favor in the presence of this man (Nehemiah 1:11).***

Your pastor has many demands on his time and will undoubtedly want to know what you need him to do with respect to this new ministry. Remember, his job is not to manage the nursing home ministry. He is called to equip, support or facilitate lay ministry **(Ephesians 4:11-12)**. We recommend you:

- Ask your pastor to pray for you and to encourage other church members to join you either in ministry or intercessory prayer. This kind of pastoral support will be most helpful and encouraging to all the team members.

- Be sure your pastor understands that you and the team are willing to do the actual work of the ministry, but welcome him to participate as often as he may desire. Some pastors really enjoy and have a special gift for nursing home ministry. Some might want to be involved on a regular basis, but others will be happy to delegate responsibility to you.

- Ask for an opportunity to present the ministry to the congregation as a whole, preferably at a time when the pastor is also present, for example, during a Sunday morning service. One good time is during National Nursing Home Week, which falls on the week of Mother's Day each year.

- The pastor will be concerned that you are not taking on more than you are capable of handling. Your pastor may recommend you set some limitations; be submissive and faithful and *"Don't despise the day of small things" (Zechariah 4:10)*. Soon you will have many more open doors.

- Don't drag the meeting with the pastor out past the scheduled time. You should be able to make this presentation in a half hour.

- Be prepared to take notes from your pastor's instructions and opinions.

- Express gratitude for your pastor's support and leadership.

Follow-up

- Once plans have been formulated for the nursing-home ministry, write them up and submit them to your pastor for review, approval and support.

- After the nursing-home ministry gets underway, you will want to update your pastor periodically either personally or by a letter or report. It is very normal for pastors not to know the full details of your ministry; therefore, you cannot assume your pastor will know when you are having problems. Many pastors work from the no-news-is-good-news policy, so let him know the good and the bad news.

RECRUITING CHURCH MEMBERS

Your next step will be to recruit church members for the care team. As described in detail in Chapter 6, a care team is usually made up of four to six people who will focus on one nursing home near your church. We recommend that you start with one team, even if you recruit as many as ten volunteers, because it is not uncommon for some to drop out of the ministry after a few visits.

Remember when recruiting help, that you are asking people to give one of life's most valued resources: TIME. Volunteers need to sense that there is an immediate and important need and a specific plan to meet the need. Proper preparation, presentation, and follow-up are essential.

Preparation

You will need to prepare to give your church a brief but very clear picture of the need, the Biblical rationale for the ministry, and specific ways church members can meet these needs. It is most helpful to include a short testimony or two of a recent ministry blessing. Experienced nursing-home missionaries from other churches may be a great support; they can pray with and for you and help you prepare. If you have already been visiting and have established some relationships with Christians in a nursing home, you may also want to ask them to pray for this ministry.

You should have a way for people who are interested in the ministry to sign up. A flyer in your church bulletin can include a place for them to print their name and phone number. This could be dropped in the offering or left at the church office. Be sure your own name and phone number are on the flyer, as some will want to pray before they commit. The Sonshine Society has an informative flyer that can be put in your church bulletin. This printed material can include details that you may not have time to cover during your presentation. (See our Resource Chapter).

Presentation

Your presentation should be upbeat, Biblically based, and encouraging. Focus on the positive ways people can minister to nursing-home residents, not the obstacles. Avoid manipulation and using guilt as a motivator. Let the facts about the need for ministry speak for themselves. Your presentation should be only as long as the time given you. If you are told, "Take four to five minutes," take only four to five minutes. Your pastor will appreciate your submission.

To help you organize your thoughts for a five-minute presentation, we provide an example of what could be included. Feel free to use it "as is," or modify it as needed:

- Good morning!
- In John 4:35, Jesus said, "Do you not say, 'Four months more and then the harvest'? I tell you, open your eyes and look at the fields! They are ripe for harvest."
- I would like to tell you about a mission field that is very ripe and awaiting harvesters. It does not require you to go overseas or even out of state; it is right here in our community.
- Approximately ___ miles from our church there is a nursing home called ___. There are approximately ___ people who live there. Many are very lonely and some are near death; some are Christians and others have never established a personal relationship with Jesus. Because of the 20-month turnover, there will be approximately _____ other people living there within two years.
- Nursing-home residents have the same needs as all of us. One primary need is for Christian fellowship that will help them to find hope and peace in Jesus.
- One problem nursing-home residents have that people outside the nursing home don't have is they are not able to leave the nursing home to fellowship with other believers in a church of their choice.

- The church must take the initiative, be intentional, and go to the nursing home.
- It only takes about six people to create a care team that can adopt this home. By providing spiritual refreshment to nursing-home residents on a regular basis, we may prevent many of these folks from dying of spiritual malnutrition.
- Some of you may be asking the Lord what kind of ministry He wants you to honor Him in. Please consider the nursing-home ministry.
- The Bible says in Matthew 25:40, "The King will reply, 'I tell you the truth, whatever you did for one of the least of these brothers of mine, you did for me.'" In verses 35 and 36 Jesus said, "For I was hungry and you gave me something to eat, I was thirsty and you gave me something to drink, I was a stranger and you invited me in, I needed clothes and you clothed me, I was sick and you looked after me, I was in prison and you came to visit me."
- The Bible also says in James 1:27, "Religion that God our Father accepts as pure and faultless is this: to look after orphans and widows in their distress…"
- It is quite clear that it is not the responsibility of the nursing home to meet the spiritual needs of these neighbors of ours. It is God's will that the church embrace this responsibility.
- It is also clearly part of our church's vision to:___ (here you can quote the portion of your church's vision that would include ministry to nursing homes).
- Not only can a nursing-home care team be a blessing to the people living in the nursing home; there are also many volunteers who have told us their lives were transformed by being on a nursing-home ministry care team.

- On (date) we will be conducting a half-day workshop to establish a care team to minister in this home.
- The workshop will include an overview of nursing-home ministry and a trip to the nursing home for orientation. Following the nursing home visit, we will return to the church for a light lunch and share our experiences and plan for the future.
- I have come today to invite you to consider joining this ministry team. I speak on behalf of those who cannot speak for themselves. Come to the workshop and see how you can be used of the Lord to give Him a drink through a few thirsty people in our community.
- _____ and I will be here after the service to talk further with you and give you a flyer with all the details.
- May the Lord bless and guide you in your decisions.

You can see from the above example that there are three main points:
1. There is a great need.
2. There is a specific plan to meet the need.
3. Any Christian that wants to serve the Lord can be part of the care team.

Whether you use our example or develop your own, we recommend you clearly address these three points. Also, be sure to share one or two pertinent Scriptures to validate your overall message. We would further suggest that when you give your presentation, share from your heart; and avoid preaching or using gimmicks to convince your audience. You want people who are going to respond from their heart, not as a result of compulsion or manipulation. You need to be confident that the Lord of the Harvest has heard your prayers to send forth the workers for the harvest **(Matthew 9:36-38).**

Videos, slide presentations, skits and testimonies are all possible avenues of presentation. Note: Throughout the years of using videos in our training programs, we have discovered that small screens and fuzzy pictures are usually counterproductive. Therefore, use the largest size video projection and the highest-quality equipment possible.

It is normal for churches to allow you only one ministry presentation a year, and in some cases it may not be possible at all. Large churches that have multiple services on Sunday morning do not always afford the time to give a presentation. For this and other reasons, your pastor may not permit a presentation to be given to the whole church. Arrangements might be made, however, for you to share with a Sunday School class or some of the church's smaller fellowship groups, like a seniors' ministry or young couples' ministry. Another alternative could be to have the pastor make an announcement about the nursing-home ministry for a few weeks in succession and invite members to an after-service pizza luncheon/presentation. Your pastor should come to this meeting, at least, to give the opening welcome and prayer. His presence will express his support and will also help draw members. Include information about this meeting in the church bulletin.

Consider National Nursing Home Week (the week of Mother's Day) as a good time for presenting this opportunity. Your pastor may also welcome *seed planting efforts,* such as an informative bulletin board or poster with your phone number on it. An encouraging testimony in the church newsletter or brief comment in the weekly bulletin may keep the opportunity to serve visible. Be prayerful and creative and enjoy your labor of faith.

Our experience has shown that the most effective way of recruiting help is after the church is aware of the nursing home ministry. People can also be invited on an individual basis. Words like, "Come and see if this is the ministry which the Lord would have you share in," have worked well. You can offer to give them a ride for the first few visits. The fellowship on the way to the home can be a great way to build a good relationship.

Follow-up

Your willingness to follow up on a potential team member is very important. Follow-up is essential for the longevity of the ministry. Many people will be touched by a good presentation and may want to try the ministry. However, they may have concerns that need to be addressed. Some of the possible concerns include:

- fear of getting into an awkward situation and not knowing what to do
- fears that they might say or do the wrong thing
- feeling that they have no special talents and therefore have nothing to give

Some people may not even be able to verbalize these concerns, but if we are good listeners, we will be able to pick up on some of these fears and feelings of inadequacy, and offer helpful insights to encourage them to take steps of faith. Remember, our enemy the devil whispers words of doubt and fear to try to stop all of us, but grace, truth and mutual encouragement will overpower him.

> *You are asking people to give one of life's most valued resources: Time. The potential team members will need to sense that there is a viable need and a specific plan to meet the need.*

When a person is asked to volunteer, he should be told what specific tasks are involved, approximately how much time is needed for the ministry, and what benefits he can expect. An effort should be made to allow each volunteer some choice of activities and to tailor tasks to meet the individual's skills and interests.

Some thought should be given to the circumstances of potential volunteers. Are there mothers with young children at home? More volunteers would be forthcoming if babysitting was available while they minister at the nursing home; they also might consider bringing their children to the nursing home. If the volunteers themselves are elderly, they may need transportation to enable them to become involved. If youth groups are involved, activities will need to be scheduled in the late afternoon and early evening hours. Some people may not be able to actually go to the nursing home but would be willing to give administrative help, provide transportation or childcare. Try to involve every willing servant.

These general guidelines for follow-up may also be helpful:

- Be prepared to share your experiences regarding the ministry.
- Be cheerful, polite, and encouraging. Your zeal will be contagious.
- Be prayerful and trust the Lord of the Harvest to send forth laborers.
- Be a servant leader who is willing to go the extra mile when necessary.
- Generally, if a person does not respond after three calls, and perhaps a letter, it's an indication they are not yet ready to commit to this type of ministry.
- According to **1 Corinthians 12** and **Romans 12,** every Christian has at least one gift to share for the common good of others. However, many Christians avoid getting involved with ministry because they do not believe they have much to offer. A little encouragement and support often causes these timid servants to blossom and flourish.
- Always have a plan with concrete principles and guidelines to get started. It is also important to welcome creative suggestions from team members.
- Although you may desire many team members, the Lord may provide only one. Consider the value of one faithful team member. Paul said of Timothy, *"I have no one else like him, who takes a genuine interest in your*

welfare. For everyone looks out for his own interests, not those of Jesus Christ. But you know that Timothy has proved himself, because as a son with his father he has served with me in the work of the gospel." (Philippians 2:20-22)

- Be faithful and grateful with small things and small beginnings; the Lord will give you many more opportunities for service in the future.

CARE-TEAM TRAINING

Whatever approach you choose, we recommend that each team member receive some initial form of training. There are many ways to provide this. The Sonshine Society has a very helpful training video that includes a great format for both one-to-one and group ministry. Be sure to allow time during the training for questions and comments. You might invite the Activities Director of the home where you will be visiting (to your training session) to share other practical ways volunteers can assist in the nursing home. It is useful to do some role-playing so that volunteers can participate in simulated situations similar to those they may actually encounter. If possible, have the new team members work alongside a more experienced member. When possible, the experienced members can patiently delegate simple responsibilities to enable the inexperienced to learn and grow.

It is also profitable to provide each volunteer with a written description of what he is expected to do, and the team leader's phone number if there is a need to cancel or if the new volunteer has questions. A volunteer commitment statement can be a useful tool for specifying basic responsibilities and expectations. See appendix for an example of a "Volunteer Questionnaire".

KEEPING THE TEAM TOGETHER

It should be expected that a certain percentage of volunteers who begin with great enthusiasm will drop out shortly after they start. There are many reasons for this including: a change in one's personal situation which makes volunteering impossible, a misunderstanding of what was required, or anxiety about one's performance. In most cases, the volunteer can be made more comfortable if assigned to a different task.

Plan to follow up with all new volunteers, particularly those whose enthusiasm seems to be lagging. It is better to ask, "What can I do to enable you to return?" than to pressure them and make them feel guilty. Sometimes, a bit of personal support is all that is needed. Let the Lord convict. Your role as a leader, and the role of the more experienced team members, is to encourage.

After a person has begun work as a volunteer, he must not be taken for granted. We find it extremely profitable to invest time in building personal as well as team relationships. Jesus modeled this, as He would often withdraw to spend time alone with His disciples. Relationships need to be cultivated and nurtured. Below are some tips for nurturing your team relationships:

- Encourage team members by spending time with them aside from the time spent in the nursing homes. Encourage them with cards, an occasional phone call, or a meeting over coffee. Plan a monthly or bi-monthly luncheon for the team to express your appreciation to team members.

- Pray for your team members. Be aware of their needs and tell them that you are praying for them.

- Remember that teams that visit weekly in one nursing home stay together longer than those who visit several homes monthly.

- Provide support meetings for open discussion, topical instruction, the sharing of experiences and any prayer requests. These meetings will give the team an opportunity to communicate concerns and desires. Their input is very important.

- Be a servant. If a person stops going to a nursing home, instead of asking why and pressuring him to come back, sensitively explore the reasons for dropping out and, if possible, eliminate obstacles by providing any needed support. Some people may need to drop out of the ministry for a season only and then return when family or personal circumstances permit.

- Be willing to make adjustments and changes as team members offer suggestions that might enhance the team's effectiveness.

- Invest time to learn the strengths of various team members and use them in ministry. Step back so others can step forward. People flourish best when they minister using their gifts and strengths. (This does not mean, however, we will never have to do things we do not like to do.)

- It is a blessing to know we are dependent on and appreciated by each other.

- Accountability is important but effective only when team members have previously understood and agreed on what is expected of them.

- A volunteer appreciation/recognition program can be a great source of encouragement. Articles in the church newsletter, bulletin board displays, years-of-service pins, or gifts during special annual luncheons or dinners, are all possible ways of building up the faithful care-team servants. Most Christians do not minister for praise or rewards; however, all Christians appreciate being thanked and valued by their friends. Honor people for work well done, with all sincerity.

> **Whoever serves me must follow me; and where I am, my servant also will be. My Father will honor the one who serves me.**
>
> **John 12:26**
>
> **Be devoted to one another in brotherly love. Honor one another above yourselves.**
>
> **Romans 12:10**

NURSING HOME MINISTRY SEEDS

You may find it necessary to convince fellow Christians and even church leaders of the importance and responsibility of having a nursing-home ministry, even after the ministry is well under way. Everyone will not be as committed as you are. Be careful not to take rejection personally. It is the Lord who sends forth the workers. Seeds planted in soil prepared by the Lord can produce fruit bearing trees; be careful not to contaminate the ground with resentment. *For man's anger does not bring about the righteous life that God desires (James 1:20).*

We recommend the following reasons as possible seeds of encouragement. They could be included in church bulletins or as you speak to others about the ministry. Remember, you may need to continually or periodically bring this need up before the congregation. As you share each point verbally or through a church bulletin, try to include a practical example from the nursing home ministry to illustrate the point being made.

1. Jesus both desires and commands that we reach out in love to those who are less fortunate than we are. *And this is his command: to believe in the name of his Son,*

Jesus Christ, and to love one another as he commanded us (1 John 3:23).

2. Many people in nursing homes are starving for Christian fellowship. *My friends and companions avoid me because of my wounds; my neighbors stay far away (Psalm 38:11).*

3. If we were in a place where we could not get out to go to church, we would want others to bring the church to us. *If you really keep the royal law found in Scripture, "Love your neighbor as yourself," you are doing right (James 2:8).*

4. Nursing-home ministry gives us the opportunity to touch the very heart of God. *"The King will reply, `I tell you the truth, whatever you did for one of the least of these brothers of mine, you did for me'" (Matthew 25:40).*

5. Nursing-home ministry gives Christians who desire to serve God -- but believe they have little or nothing to offer -- a chance to discover that they truly do have much to offer. *There are different kinds of gifts, but the same Spirit. There are different kinds of service, but the same Lord. There are different kinds of working, but the same God works all of them in all men. Now to each one the manifestation of the Spirit is given for the common good. All these are the work of one and the same Spirit, and He gives them to each one, just as He determines (1 Corinthians 12:4-7 & 11).*

6. Nursing-home ministry gives the church an opportunity to be a witness of Christ's character in its own community. *"By this all men will know that you are my disciples, if you love one another." (John 13:35).*

> Not every Christian is called to minister in a nursing home, but every Christian church should have an outreach to at least one care center in their community.

7. If each church would faithfully and consistently reach out to just one nursing home, the people living there would not die of spiritual malnutrition! There are approximately 20,000 skilled-care nursing homes and more then 350,000 churches in North America. Over two thousand people die in nursing homes each day, many without a friend to hold their hand. *Religion that God our Father accepts as pure and faultless is this: to look after orphans and widows in their distress and to keep oneself from being polluted by the world (James 1:27).*

8. A properly established nursing-home ministry care team can impact over sixty people each week; and it is one of the least expensive ministries to maintain. *It is like a mustard seed, which is the smallest seed you plant in the ground. Yet when planted, it grows and becomes the largest of all garden plants, with such big branches that the birds of the air can perch in its shade" (Mark 4:31-32).*

9. It is wrong for us to know of people in our community who are in such desperate need and turn our backs on them. *Anyone, then, who knows the good he ought to do and doesn't do it, sins (James 4:17).*

10. When a church's outreach program is rooted primarily in the desire to increase its membership, it is giving to get something in return. Reaching out only to potential members is not necessarily rooted in charity. Christians who reach out in a spirit of love come to a deeper relationship with God, because God is love. *Dear friends, let us love one another, for love comes from God. Everyone who loves has been born of God and knows God. Whoever does not love does not know God, because God is love. . .Whoever lives in love lives in God, and God in him (1 John 4:7-8 &16b).*

DO'S & DON'TS FOR RECRUITING VOLUNTEERS

The following recruiting guidelines are a summary of this chapter and also a quick checklist to assist you in your recruiting efforts:

Do's

- **Pray** that the Lord of the Harvest will send the workers.
- **Be creative.** Some people feel they have nothing to offer because they cannot preach, sing or evangelize. Explain that there are many other areas of need. Be organized and prepared to have team members engage in small tasks so they can see that they are truly needed. Examples include: taking attendance at services, gathering residents for services, turning pages of songbooks, and friendly visitation following the service. See also "The Ministry Care Team's Role" in Chapter 6.
- **Share fresh testimonies** with your church about what God has done in the nursing home that you visit.
- **Share prayer requests** of residents you visit with your nursing home ministry team. Sometimes resident prayer requests may also be shared at a church prayer meeting, but you need to be concerned with issues of **confidentiality**. Don't share specific names of people in the nursing home, specific health issues or names of family members. If a resident has requested prayer, it would be appropriate also to ask him if you have permission to share that need and with what group of people.
- **Encourage family involvement** in the Nursing Home Ministry. Many residents love to have children and also pets visit.

- **Plant seeds.** Copy articles from nursing-home-ministry newsletters and put them in the church bulletin or give the newsletters to potential volunteers.
- **Be relational.** Involve yourself with your church in small but important ways that will enable you to meet and serve other members. Your humble and faithful service in other areas of the church will earn you respect and greater influence when you present your request to the church.

> *The kingdom of God is built and advances through relationships.*

- **Seek and foster relationships with other nursing home ministries.** In addition to your pastor's support, we recommend you contact and, if possible, fellowship with other successful nursing-home-ministry teams in area churches.
- **Focus on one nursing home in your community:** Teams that visit weekly in one nursing home normally stay together longer and are easier to maintain than those who visit several homes monthly. If your team grows to over eight consistent members, consider splitting into two teams.
- **Establish goals.** Weekly visits to a nursing home are the desirable goal. If a volunteer is not able to visit weekly, welcome whatever time he can give and pray for possible adjustments that may enable him to achieve the goal.
- **Encourage a commitment.** Ask the new volunteer to commit to four visits before he decides to drop out or stay with the team. (Several people have started in nursing-home ministry thinking it was only a temporary ministry; then after several months, they realize that the Lord was calling them to stay.)

- **Make introductions.** On the first visit, be sure to introduce the volunteer to a few residents who are pleasant and able to express appreciation for the visit.
- **Be patient and reaffirming.** New volunteers may do things or say things that are improper. If possible, do not correct them in front of others. Be reaffirming as you instruct.
- **Encourage.** Plan to spend a few minutes with new volunteers before leaving the nursing home, to answer any questions and sharing blessings/concerns. You may need to include a time of prayer for the Lord to help overcome obstacles.
- **Recognize.** Hold periodic volunteer appreciation/recognition events to honor and bless the faithful servants.
- **Build a solid foundation.** Lasting growth builds on a good foundation. When we are not prepared, the Lord may not bring more help. When we are prepared and faithful with a little, the increase will come because it is our Father's will that we bear much fruit.
- **Aspire for Quality.** The Lord is concerned with quality control. Remember, we labor in His name!

Don'ts

- **Put a guilt trip on potential volunteers or pressure them.** Be gentle and respectful, and understand that not everyone is called to nursing-home ministry.
- **Ask initially for too great a time commitment.** Encourage potential volunteers to come along with you and see what you do. God is faithful and He will let them know if the nursing home ministry is where He wants them.

- **Ask for volunteers if you do not have a specific way to get them involved.** Many potential team members go elsewhere because they feel there is no real need for them.

Again, I tell you that if two of you on earth agree about anything you ask for, it will be done for you by my Father in heaven. For where two or three come together in my name, there am I with them (Matthew 18:19-20).

As you go forth to recruit team members, you need not be shy. You are inviting people to participate with our Heavenly Father in a great mission field. As you have been blessed in this ministry, those who accept the invitation will most likely be blessed. Indeed, you are inviting them to invest into heavenly treasures, which last forever.

> Do not store up for yourselves treasures on earth, where moth and rust destroy, and where thieves break in and steal. But store up for yourselves treasures in heaven, where moth and rust do not destroy, and where thieves do not break in and steal. For where your treasure is, there your heart will be also (Matthew 6:19-21).

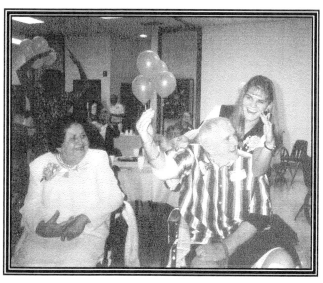

Clap your hands, all you nations; shout to God with cries of joy

(Psalm 47:1).

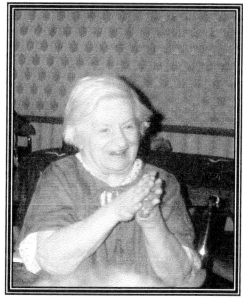

CHAPTER 10

SPECIAL SERVICES AND ACTIVITIES

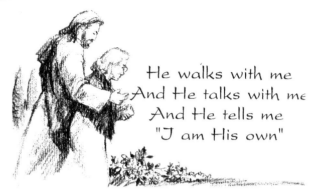

He walks with me
And He talks with me
And He tells me
"I am His own"

"Even when I am old and gray, do not forsake me, O God, till I declare your power to the next generation, your might to all who are to come" (Psalm 71:18).

As emphasized throughout this book, our primary mission is to share the love and Word of God through caring relationships in nursing homes. There are many creative ways to accomplish our mission in addition to the one-to-one visits and church services modeled in previous chapters. Missionaries throughout the world are bearing fruit through many special services and activities. They share both their spiritual and their natural gifts in practical ways, meeting basic or essential needs of the people whom they are sent to serve. Some of these activities are religious or spiritual in nature, while some are not. But all of them still have the same ultimate goal: sharing Jesus Christ.

There may be people in your church who are not able to visit in a nursing home on a regular basis, but would be willing to share in a special service a few times a year. In this chapter, we share stories, testimonies and practical tips of those who found creative ways to bless the residents by sharing their unique gifts and talents. These, of course, are only a few of the many possibilities. So be creative and remember: special services and extra efforts your church makes will show your friends that they are special.

COMMUNION SERVICES

During Holy Week services prior to Easter, I lead a Lord's Supper Communion Service in the nursing home. I have shared during staff training which residents physically should and should not partake. Prior to the service, the daughter of one of our residents came and asked if her mother Bea could partake. This is a resident who did not seem to have much comprehension and could not answer any questions or hold a conversation. She had not talked in months and just stared into space. I shared with the daughter that, with her assistance in helping her mother partake of the cup and bread, it might be meaningful to her. When one of our volunteers walked past Bea with the cup and bread, she reached out for the bread. She took it in her hand, focused on it, looked it over and examined it. She then took of both the cup and bread and made these comments. "Oh, I am so glad they are letting me take the Lord's Supper. It has been eight years since I have gone to my church and have partaken in the supper. And oh, how this brings back memories of childhood taking the supper in a country church. Oh thank you for letting me do this. It means so much to me. I am thankful for what Jesus has done for me on the cross." Her daughter that said for three days after the service, Bea talked about taking of the Lord's Supper. She died less than a week later. Seeing and touching the bread, and taking of the cup, helped orient her to reality. It caused her to reflect back on her life and allowed both Bea and her daughter to have very

meaningful last days. Let us not underestimate the power of remembering our Lord Jesus in Communion. Communion has no magical powers, but there is power in the presence of the Lord.
   Chaplain Chris Finley, Oklahoma Baptist Homes

Many nursing-home residents desire to receive Holy Communion. In **Deuteronomy 16:10-14**, God makes special provisions to include the widow in the covenant life of His people. Widows are to rejoice at the feasts of God *with* His people in community. These verses in Deuteronomy have implications for the presence of widows (and elderly) at the Lord's Supper, the New Testament feast of God.

Nursing home residents are often overlooked in this area of the church's spiritual life. Perhaps a way to overcome this is to work with the Director of Activities and ask residents to indicate their desire to receive communion. Offer to help arrange for their pastor (sometimes a lay minister) to come on a scheduled basis to share in it. If possible, you may want to accompany the minister to provide a link to your group services in the home. Churches should also be encouraged to transport their own members who are nursing-home residents to their communion services.

In some cases, clergy support may not be available to meet the individual needs of all the residents. You may, instead, choose to hold a communion service yourself. Since there are many theological and denominational differences and concerns regarding the meaning and method of sharing Holy Communion, it is important to reconcile these by prayerfully reading the Scriptures and seeking your pastor's counsel. Understanding the different perspectives from other churches represented in the home can help you be sensitive to all.

If you are not able to resolve your own concerns, we recommend you do not have communion services. If you choose to, however, the following guidelines may help:

Suggested model for Communion services

It is important to work out a dignified and comfortable routine so the service is free from awkward mistakes or violations of common Biblical practices. A service structure could be as follows:

- Opening prayer
- A few songs of worship
- A Scripture reading
- A brief devotional
- Presenting the Bread and Wine (Grape juice is generally used and very thin communion wafers that dissolve in the mouth can help prevent any choking)
- General instructions
- The minister distributes the elements (perhaps with the assistance of others), while the rest are being led in songs of worship and praise. This can take time if there are many residents who need help; please don't rush.
- After all are served, a closing Scripture and/or song
- Benediction

Other points regarding communion:

- There are some concerns about residents choking on the bread (or wafer). Some ministers dip the bread in the cup saying, "The body and blood of our Lord Jesus given out of love and mercy for you." Then they carefully place the juice-soaked bread into the resident's mouth without touching them. Be sure to also carry a napkin for possible spills.

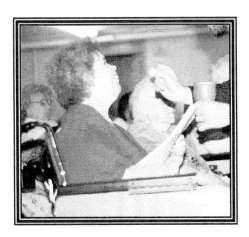

- As mentioned above, staff involvement can be a great help to you, and a great blessing for themselves as well.

- In services that have more than twenty residents, it is helpful to have a song leader leading familiar worship songs that would require minimal page turning, thus minimizing helper movement around the room.

- Some denominations allow only the Pastor to serve communion. This could be a good opportunity to invite him occasionally to share in your nursing-home outreach. It will bless him and the residents.

- Communion is for all Christians, but some Christians do not have peace about receiving it from a minister of a different denomination or from a layperson. It is important to inform the residents that all Christians are welcome to receive, *in remembrance of Jesus.* However, if for any reason they do not want to, they may indicate by saying, "No thank you," when you or the minister comes by. It is important for us not to make residents feel uncomfortable when they decline.

- Ministers' service manuals provide additional guidance for such services.

- Remember, too, that communion may be given to people individually at their bedside, if they are unable to come to the service itself. Be very careful when administering this in bed; a person's head should be elevated some to prevent choking. Always make sure the person has swallowed all of the bread or wafer before you leave the room. You might ask a nurse or nursing assistant to accompany you. You could begin by sharing Scripture and end with a brief prayer.

A MOBILE GOSPEL TEAM

An effective way for care teams to share the love and Word of God with bed-bound residents is through a *mobile gospel team*. The mission of this team is to provide a mini church service for those who cannot attend group worship services. The team is usually made up of three to five members who visit various rooms to give a mini worship service. The order of service may vary a little according to the different needs of each resident you visit. As noted above, communion may also be given through this gospel team to bed-bound or room-bound residents. The following is one helpful model for visiting as a team:

Suggested model for a Mobile Gospel Team

- A brief introduction: A greeting, with a reminder of the purpose for the visit.
- Opening prayer
- A song, with an offer to sing one of the resident's favorites.
- A two - three minute sermonette/devotional
- A prayer time including any personal requests
- A benediction
- An opportunity for the resident to ask questions or talk
- A polite exit

This simple little format has been used quite effectively, and residents will often ask you to return. The team can minister in ten to fifteen rooms in about two hours. Each visit takes between five and seven minutes.

RESIDENTS IN MINISTRY

*A few years ago, I (Bill) became increasingly aware that the Christian residents were enjoying our Bible studies, but they were not being active in their faith. I was concerned, because I knew that their faith without deeds of love was less than God's will for them. After praying about this, I decided to invite the more physically able and cognitively-intact residents to meet with me on another day of the week to address this concern. I explained to them how I was concerned for the residents that were not willing or able to come to the services. I also explained that I was not able to visit all of these unchurched people and needed help to do so. I further shared Scriptures to encourage them to be active in their faith and challenged them to give the Lord an hour or so of their day to care for fellow residents **(1John 3:16-18, James 2:14-17, Galatians 5:6b).** All seven of these residents expressed a willingness to serve the Lord, so I presented the following ministry outreach which we later called the Love Your Neighbor Ministry:*

Love your neighbor ministry

Our purpose:

To help our neighbors (fellow nursing-home residents) by encouraging them with the love and Word of God.

Our goal:

To be a faithful friend to at least two of our neighbors who do not have many visitors or seem to be discouraged.

Our method:

To visit daily or on a regular basis to encourage and cheer. When appropriate, to offer inspiring Bible verses and a short prayer.
Most important: just be a friend and show that you care, reminding them that Jesus loves them.

Before we visit:

We pray for our friends, asking the LORD to use us to love them in Jesus' name.

Follow-up:

Each week we gather to share experiences (not gossip) and pray for our friends.

Occasionally I give each of our visiting residents large print Scripture verses that they can share with their friends. Our weekly follow-up time would also include testimonies, prayer requests, personal reflections, and Bible questions. Sometimes I share a short devotional.

This ministry took off very slowly and continues to require a lot of enthusiasm, encouragement and patient coaching. The residents, however, remain faithful in their daily visits, as long as they feel well enough to get out of their rooms. As the years roll on, we have had to say good-bye to most of our original team, but new team members have enabled the ministry to continue.

This labor of love has been fruitful. Some of the benefits have been:
- The visiting residents have become more active in their faith and less focused on their own personal troubles.
- Several lonely residents now have a friend who visits them several times each week.
- Because we've met almost weekly, we have gotten to know each other better and appreciate each other more.
- Most of the active residents have learned to openly ask important spiritual questions and have led in prayer during our meetings.
- The atmosphere of the home has become much more friendly and adaptable for new residents.

In another nursing home, I (Bill) started another team with a little different approach. Along with an open Bible study, I encouraged residents to do at least one good deed each day. We are just starting, and are finding some progress already. I find that these residents need a lot of encouragement too, as they feel they have little or nothing to offer. They need tiny tasks to get them started. Once they get started, they progress and discover that the Lord can use them to do much good. Their lives are greatly enhanced, and so is the overall atmosphere of the home.

What some residents are doing to be active in their faith:
- Sit in the main lobby and greet people when they come to the home.
- Help put bibs on residents during meals. (Bibs also can be accompanied by a friendly hug.)
- Help turn pages of hymn books during church services.
- Take attendance for church service. This person can also remind team members if they forgot to bring someone.
- Play the Bible on tape for a small group or for an individual resident.

- Pray for care team and area pastors. One man asked a pastor for one prayer request each week. The pastor relied on this man as a great source of support.
- Visit new residents to welcome them to the home and invite them to the weekly Bible study and church service.

Lying in a nursing-home rehab bed surrounded by modesty curtains on two sides and windows on the other side, our friend Katie shared with us the following story: One day a resident whom she didn't know wheeled herself into Katie's room, coming in around the curtain at the foot of the bed. "Hello there!" said Katie, and the lady warmly smiled a return greeting. They chatted about nothing in particular for a while, and then Katie said to this gray-haired lady, "Do you know Jesus?" Katie tells that, at the name of Jesus, this lady quickly turned to leave the room, even tangling her wheelchair up in the curtains in her attempt to exit.

A few days later, again the unnamed resident came to see Katie-behind-the-curtains and conversed very comfortably about the weather and each other's health, until Katie asked again if she knew Jesus. Again, the lady quickly turned to leave the room, with the curtains again getting tangled in the spokes of her wheel chair. Eventually she freed herself and raced out of the room.

The same thing happened a third time--and a fourth. Finally, on the fifth visit, the lady gathered her courage and when Katie asked if she knew Jesus, she replied, "Well, I know ABOUT Him, but I don't KNOW Him." "Would you like to?" Katie asked and the little lady in the wheelchair almost whispered, "Yes, I really would!" So Katie led her through the steps up to the throne of grace.

Shortly after, Katie was transferred to another care center. It seems that the Lord had assigned this task specifically for Katie, and when she had completed it, He moved her on. Perhaps to the next assignment.

Marilyn Barrett

The righteous will flourish like a palm tree, they will grow like a cedar of Lebanon; planted in the house of the LORD, they will flourish in the courts of our God. They will still bear fruit in old age, they will stay fresh and green, proclaiming, "The LORD is upright; he is my Rock, and there is no wickedness in him." (Psalm 92:12-15)

CHILDREN AND YOUTH IN THE NURSING HOME

About two years ago, I joined a Care Team that conducts a Tuesday afternoon worship service at a local nursing home. A woman on the team told me she had been trying every week, without success, to get Clinton to come to worship. She suggested that, as a man, I might have more success in relating to Clinton. Well, the short story is, I didn't. Although Clinton always welcomed me when I stopped by his room, he consistently had a reason why he could not, at that moment, come to our service.

About a year later, God used another vessel to reach out to Clinton. Nancy had come to our service on occasion during the past year. One day Nancy brought her grandson Seth and they stopped by to visit Clinton. During the visit, Seth invited Clinton to come to our worship service and he responded with a firm "Yes."

> *This was the first time I had ever seen Clinton outside of his room, and what a feeling of excitement I had! Following our service I asked Seth if he would escort Clinton back to his room. I also thanked Clinton for coming, and asked if I could count on him being with us in the weeks ahead. He said yes.*
>
> *Isn't it amazing how the Lord sent a five-year-old child to do in one visit what others could not accomplish in over a year. Praise be to God for his servants of all ages!*
>
> Bob McGregor

The nursing home is a mission field in which the whole family can participate, regardless of age. One of the greatest treasures in a nursing home is the presence of children. Residents usually love and appreciate them coming to visit. Most children, once they are acquainted with the environment and with a few residents, also love the opportunity to visit. They also learn to give, to respect seniors, and to recognize their own mortality. The following is an excerpt taken from Sonshine Society's training guide, *All The Days of My Life:*

> *Florence began to visit a man, whom she had known and ministered with in former years, who had moved into a nearby care center. As this man's health failed, he became increasingly unresponsive, eventually giving no response at all. In Florence's words, "The Lord spoke to my heart saying, 'He loved children.'" The next visit, Florence brought her two-and-a-half-year-old granddaughter Jennifer. Not only did Jennifer light up the life of this unresponsive man, but also "brightened the day" for all those with whom she came in contact.*
>
> *That was nearly six years ago. The clear message of what a child's presence can do in a nursing home was not lost on Florence.*

Granddaughter Jennifer still accompanies her, and they have shared the joy of this ministry with other children and mothers in their neighborhood. The result? Today they have a pool of 15-20 youngsters and four young mothers who visit the care center. Florence goes every week, sometimes twice, sometimes three times. They go in small, well-supervised groups and are very sensitive to both staff and residents. Florence says that children often intuitively know just what to do if something out of the ordinary occurs. Although she doesn't recommend the hyperactive child for this, she says a nursing-home situation brings out the best in children.

And what about the children? Is it a drag or drudgery for them? NO WAY! They are eager to go and actually press the issue, saying, "When can we go again?"

"We often went to see ninety-nine-year-old Grandpa J. How the children loved to sing and hug Grandpa J. and, always, he was so responsive. Then one day, Grandpa J. really went to higher care. His memorial service was held. I went to the son after the service saying how much the children loved his father. The son brought tears to my eyes as he said, "One of the last things Dad said, just hours before he died, was how much he loved to have the children come."

One of our mothers had a baby and now she takes the tiny one to the rest home. The delight experienced is exciting!

And then there is Wing D. This area is a locked unit to prevent the residents from wandering away. Twenty-nine precious Grandmas and Grandpas are there, most in varying stages of dementia. I hesitated even going into that area, but over five years ago, a mom who was with me suggested we should. I asked, "Why?" And she said, "I used to work at this nursing home. This is a favorite place to work. Let's go." So we went.

Through the years, the children ASK to go to the "locked room"— how can they understand? But there is NEVER a moment of misbehavior there. The children have such compassion for their friends. It is there we sing action choruses, "Some Folks Want to March in the Infantry," and "Rolled Away," and "King of Kings." Sometimes the residents say, "Sing it again!" One big surprise was that some could join in singing "Jesus Loves Me" and "Oh, How I Love Jesus," but couldn't carry on a conversation at all. A man who worked there said to me, "After the children have left Wing D, the atmosphere has changed." All praise to God!

Does it pay to go to the rest home once a week, and sometimes two or three times? It pays MORE than I ever dreamed it would! The mothers tell me it has given their children a great love and respect for the elderly wherever they meet them! It is giving me the joy of working with these "younger wives," having our home filled with the laughter of the children as they come here after visitation for treats, and to have fun with their friends.

Herm Haakenson & Florence Turnidge,
All the Days of My Life

Tips on children and youth in nursing-home ministry

- You may want to introduce nursing-home outreach through special school or social projects.
- Youth and children can be great helpers for gathering residents, distributing songbooks and finding pages during the service. They also make great friends.
- Group gatherings allow young (and old) people to exercise their faith and develop their natural and spiritual gifts.

- Having the youth visit once or twice before they have their group activity can help them be more comfortable with the nursing-home environment. This will make it easier for them to focus more on the resident needs.
- Allow time to ask the youth/children questions or for them to ask questions and share experiences after their first or second visit.
- If you decide to have the youth/children share in special group presentations, encourage them to speak loudly, slowly and clearly so that residents can understand. The use of a sound system will greatly enhance the quality of sharing.
- Children will sometime resist going, as one woman testifies:

    Sometimes I care for three young children while their parents are at work. On the days that I go to the nursing home, they complain because they do not want to go. Sometimes, on the way into the home, they drag their feet and look at the floor. But suddenly one of the residents will reach out to them because they're so glad to see someone young. The children respond by reaching out to them. It is beautiful! I tell the children that God sees what they are doing and that He will bless them for their kindness to people who are confined. It's so very important for us to share what we have: time, love, smiles and a hand to hold.

    I thank God for the blessings of these dear children walking through the home with me. Just their presence brings a blessing to someone who is lonely.

    Mary Ann Goodrich

- Some youth or children may need a lot of encouragement along with basic instructions before and after the visits. If there is still resistance after three or four visits, it may be best to look for other areas of outreach. Again, allow children an opportunity to share any concerns. Some may have had grandparents who were nursing-home residents and died in the nursing home. They may be experiencing the need to talk about this.

- Regardless of the quality of the group program, residents will greatly appreciate having young visitors.
- One-to-one visits with younger people can involve storytelling, picture drawing, singing, photo sharing, reminiscing or comparing life as a child between now and 60 or 70 years ago.
- "Adoption" often occurs naturally when older adults and younger people come to know each other through participation in programs or friendly visiting.

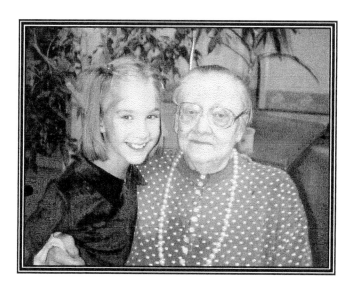

RESIDENT BIRTHDAYS

Recently, I (Bill), was told of a man who hand delivers birthday cards in a care center. After sharing the card with the resident, and talking about their birth date, he asks them about their spiritual birthday. He has led many to the Lord.

Most people appreciate being recognized on their birthday. At the beginning or end of our church services, we sing "Happy Birthday" for those recently having a birthday. Some teams present special gifts to them, for example, a box of cards or a large print book.

A birthday-card ministry can be a great tool for meeting and encouraging the residents in a nursing home. The Director of Activities would be able to supply the names and birthdays of each resident for the upcoming month. Large-print cards can be hand-made or purchased through ministries like the Sonshine Society. Be sure the print is large enough for your friend to read.

The following is an example of a birthday card with an evangelistic message; it might be appropriately used if an invitation is enclosed to the Bible studies or church services that you hold in the home.

The front of the card contains the message: "On your birthday, we want to give you the greatest gift in the world." The inside left side contains the following: "But God has already given the Greatest Gift! *For God so loved the world that he gave his one and only Son, that whoever believes in him shall not perish but have eternal life (John 3:16).* "Those who receive God's gift are born into eternal life." On the right side you can write: "Eternal Birthdays are birthed through faith in Jesus and are celebrated forever. Jesus said, "**I tell you the truth, whoever hears my word and believes him who sent me has eternal life** and will not be condemned; he has crossed over from death to life" (John 5:24).

Residents usually appreciate cards that remind them that God loves and cares for them. Cards that contain large print Psalms, like the 23rd Psalm, may be treasured. We must also consider that there is often a fine line between sharing our faith appropriately and inappropriately proselytizing. Ask the Holy Sprit to lead and guide you to the type of card to give to each resident.

MEN'S WOODSHOP

For the past six years I (Bill) have led a Men's Woodshop Class at one of the nursing homes where my wife and I also share a weekly Bible study. I was asked by the Director of Activities to give this class because most of the men would not get involved with other activities, like attending church services or Bingo. After praying, I felt a woodshop class would be a good opportunity to build relationships with the men, so I took a step of faith and accepted the challenge.

I hold two classes each month. During the first class, we assemble precut craft kits and during the second class, we paint the crafts and let the men keep them. I was able to find some woodcraft kits for less than two dollars each. The Activities Department pays for all the materials. We build cars, boats, birdhouses, airplanes, tractors and more. It is fun to see how the more capable men help those who are physically or mentally limited. We talk about experiences and tell jokes and funny stories. I also like to challenge the men by asking questions and sharing ideas that help them look to Jesus. Once I asked them, "Of all the things that make the airplane fly, what is the most important?" After several answers like "the tail," "the engine," and "the fuel," I asked, "How about the pilot? Without the pilot, the plane has no purpose but to just sit there. It would be a shame to put all the effort into building an airplane and just let it sit and rust away." After a little more discussion, I then explained, "God made us for a specific purpose; we need to let Him be the pilot of our lives or our lives will be wasted."

I used to pray that God would show me how to get the men to go to the Bible studies, because we usually had only two or three that would come. God has been good and has opened a door through the Men's Woodshop Class. Now it is unusual to have less than five men come to our church services.

Tips for having a woodshop:

- Plan for two sessions per month, usually the first and third or second and fourth week of the month. The first class is for assembling of the craft; the second class is for painting. After painting, the resident's name is put on the craft and he may keep it.
- It is difficult for one person to lead this class alone; one faithful helper is recommended.

Preparation:

- Kits can be purchased at a craft store or in larger quantities through Brandine Woodcraft Inc. 725 SW. 16th Ave., Bay #1 Delray Beach. Fl 33444, 561-266-9360.
- You may want to preassemble some parts that would be too difficult for the men to assemble; otherwise, it may take a longer time for the glue to dry before you can complete the assembly. (Experience will be your guide on this point.)

Building:

- Have the preassembled craft on the table so the men can look at it while the rest of the group is being gathered.
- Once the men are gathered, you will want to have a brief time of introductions and welcoming. This may also be a good time for a brief prayer to ask the Lord's blessing on each one present and those who could not attend; be sensitive, however, to your group. Some in the group may not initially be open to spiritual things.
- Assemble one part at a time by putting the glue in the right place and have the men mount the parts. Be sure to involve each man as much as possible. **Do not** assemble parts that they themselves can handle. Some men will take longer than others, but be patient.
- Once the craft is assembled, have the men write their names on the bottom of their craft. Tell them when you will return to have them paint it, and that they may keep the finished product.

Painting:

- The Activities Department can provide tablecloths, plastic gloves and plastic pill dispensers for the paint. One-inch foam brushes and small paint brushes for hard to reach places work best.
- Again, help only when help is needed. Some men will need you to hold the craft because they have only one working hand.
- Be prepared to do a little touch-up work.
- Give lots of honest encouragement and have fun.

This woodshop class has been very successful. Not only do the men gain a sense of purpose through woodworking, but also they have established caring friendships with one another. We believe the woodshop ministry is a reflection of Paul's challenge that we become all things to all men, so that by all possible means, we may win some to Christ **(1 Corinthians 9:19-23).**

OPENING CONVERSATIONS WITH PETS

Over the years, we have seen people bring in dogs, cats, rabbits, birds and even farm animals to visit. In some homes, animals live among the residents. As with children and singing, animals will often be the very key that causes residents to open up and talk about themselves. Occasionally, a park ranger might bring small outdoor animals from the zoo or park. This is always a highlight for residents. There are certain obvious restrictions that would apply to bringing your pets to visit, such as tags, shots, etc. You will need to ask the activities director for guidelines. Never underestimate the power of a pet for brightening the day of a nursing-home resident and for also opening up a conversation.

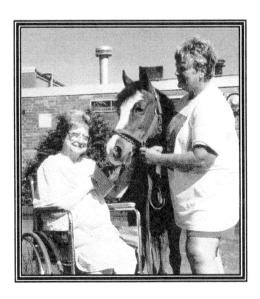

SPECIAL OUTINGS

This year our church had "Serving Others" for its Vacation Bible School theme. The leaders of VBS decided to include a servant's event for the last day of their teaching so the children could put into practice what they had learned the previous days. The servant's event was to be a day of preparing and serving a lunch for people in the community who generally lacked company or would just appreciate the fellowship. I was asked to bring residents from the local care centers.

Thankfully, I was able to have transported 28 residents from three nursing homes. These folks joined another 30 or so friends from the church and community.

We had 100 children and about 20 adult leaders each take a part. Believe it or not, it went very smoothly. The children were divided into groups of ten. Each group had a task: food preparation, serving food/drinks, special songs, skits, drama, or set-up. A group of smaller children greeted and blew bubbles at the entrance of the meeting room.

There were lots of laughs, hugs, picture taking, songs, food, and treats for all. Our friends from the nursing homes could not say enough; how they enjoyed their time away! One lady, whom I had never met before, said, "I will never forget you." Another, "This was so wonderful," and several others just said "Thank You!" many times over.

It was wonderful to see how so many children each did small tasks and caused a great blessing for many people. In closing, the emcee of the *event encouraged all of us to consider the impact on our world if each Christian did one small deed every day to bless another person, without expecting a reward. How that would impact our world around us!*

God Cares News

Outings can be a real blessing for your friends. When taking residents out of the nursing home, there is not a great need for having several activities planned. Just the opportunity to leave the building is often a complete blessing in itself. The following are ideas for places to go and things for residents to see:

- a picnic or ride in a park
- a parade
- a fair
- a ride in a car at Christmas to view lights
- a church service

Below is a testimony of one other special outing:

A few months ago, our ministry received a financial gift in memory of a friend of ours named John. John and his wife, Marian, lived in New Jersey and had made many visits in nursing homes to give cheer through music and friendly visits. A family member wanted their blessing to carry on, so with the gift came a request. "Would you do something unexpected to surprise your residents? A happy spring cake or an 'un'birthday party? Anything at all would be okay, as long as it is a break in their regular routine." What to do?? How about a picnic?? Great idea!!

The picnic came together so well. After securing an appropriate place in the park, and a bus service, we invited friends from our local nursing home. We also invited members from our church to participate, and several came to help with set-up, clean-up, cooking hot dogs, sloppy joes, potato salad, and cake. It was very easy, with almost no stress, because all the needs were shared by over a dozen volunteers who also brought music, balloons that they twisted into animals, hats, children, pets, and lots of hugs and laughs.

We are grateful for the idea and the seed of kindness. This seed will likely bear much more joy than originally anticipated, because we are planning on making this picnic an annual event.

God Cares News

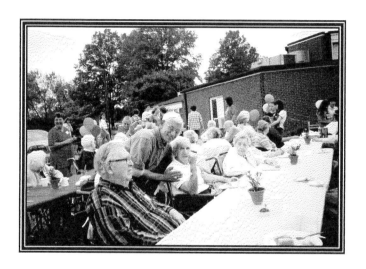

Tips on special outings:

- Try to plan a few months ahead. (Activity Directors need to plan their calendars about 5 weeks in advance.) Note also, that it is difficult for an activities director to give a specific attendance number for an outing. He may have 15 residents wanting to go, then on the day of the event some may decline because of weather, illness, mood, etc. Others may desire and ask to go for the same reasons.

- Write out details of the event for the Activities Department; i.e., location, time, theme, food (if any), person responsible, R.S.V.P. date, etc.
- If you or your church is planning on providing transportation, be sure to have a safe vehicle and proper insurance.
- Many care centers own a van with a wheelchair lift. Also, other churches in your community may have one, and be willing to be part of your special outing.
- If you are planning to take just one or two friends out in your car, be sure to have prior permission from the Activities Director before you ask your friend. You will be required to sign them out. This means you are responsible for their safety and well-being until you sign them back in.
- The Senior Adult ministry from Phoenix 1st Assembly in Arizona, has a very large "Wheelchair Bus Ministry". See our resource chapter for information on contacting them for their published materials.

CONDUCTING A VARIETY SHOW

The purpose of a variety show can be twofold: 1) to bring immediate joy and happiness through lively entertainment to nursing-home residents, staff and visitors and 2) to create an opportunity for Christians to share their love for God and faith in Christ.

You need only one committed person to start a variety show and act as a talent coordinator. This person's role is to begin by calling others and persuading them to share their talents for at least one show. You will find that your performers, after their first performance, may be quite eager to make a more long-term (even once-a-month) commitment of their time.

The talent coordinator will also be responsible for contacting the nursing home. He should contact the director of activities and set up a show time that's most convenient for all involved. If a piano is required, the coordinator will need to find out whether the home has one available. The coordinator should also call the morning of the show to remind the home of their schedule.

It is not necessary, but it may be useful in some cases, that group rehearsals occur. Each performer can practice his or her part alone, but should communicate with the coordinator about any needs for music, time and props. Leave enough time before the show to pray together and plan the order of the acts.

Find someone with an outgoing personality and a good loud speaking voice to be the Master or Mistress of Ceremonies. The emcee is a key figure, especially in adding a "spiritual note" to the show. The emcee might tell a short, humorous story with a deeper spiritual meaning. If this is told at the beginning of the show, it can be referred to at appropriate points throughout the show to reinforce the meaning.

Costuming is important. Bright, flashy colors bring joy and laughter, as does exaggerated makeup. There is no need to spend a lot of money. Sew your own costumes or have a bake sale to raise money for costumes, or buy them from thrift stores.

Older audiences enjoy many kinds of entertainment. Avoid anything that is especially "modern." Here are a few suggestions:

- Old-time sing-a-longs
- Juggling
- Banjo, harmonica, accordion, trumpet (in fact, any instrument)
- Short piano solos
- Vocal solos
- Clowns
- Tap dancing
- Soft-shoe
- Skits

A word about recruiting your talent: The acts that you are seeking are not meant to be professional. In fact, they don't have to be polished performances at all! The function of a variety show is to have fun and provide an opportunity, if you desire, to share your faith. For this reason, you should encourage interested amateurs to perform. Also, look for any opportunity for residents to participate, especially those with musical talents. Be aware of safety issues, but do not be afraid of including them. Talented staff members may also want to join you. Be aware, however, of the time factor. Keep in mind that children, too, can make a very important contribution to your show. Older people truly love to see children. Even if some of the kids are too small to participate, bring them along anyway. But be prepared—they invariably steal the show!

Having special services and activities allows volunteers to see the needs of the residents and the opportunities to make a positive difference in their lives. Just getting people to spend an hour in a nursing home will plant seeds of concern that may, one day, grow into a willingness for ongoing ministry.

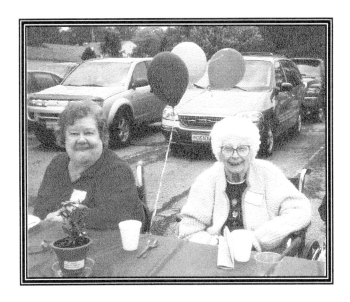

CHAPTER 11

SPECIAL ISSUES AND CONCERNS

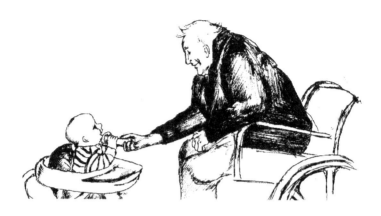

In this chapter, we are including basic information about some special issues and common concerns you might encounter while ministering in a nursing home. We will also give some helpful tips for avoiding or handling potential problems.

Because of the ever-increasing federal laws and regulations related to residents, certain issues and activities that were acceptable years ago are not permitted today. Likewise, some past activities are still acceptable but now have specific restrictions or safety requirements to be considered. Knowing and obeying the policies of the home will help assure good relations with all care-center personnel. Be sensitive to such issues and ask questions of the staff when in doubt.

PICTURE TAKING

In one of the nursing homes where I minister, there is a man who brings many blessings to several residents, family and staff. His name is

Andy. I call him "The Picture Man." Andy's wife Peg had Alzheimer's Disease, and after three years of home care and a broken hip, Andy had to choose a nursing home for her final days of care. This dedicated man, who visited Peg daily from 11:00 am until 6:30 pm, found a way to bring cheer to many others besides his wife. How? He did it with his little 35 mm camera. Andy has snapped several hundred pictures over a two-year period and has freely shared copies with those he has photographed. When I asked Andy about this, he said, "This is my ministry to these folks, my way of bringing joy and happiness to the folks here."

It is not uncommon to see some of these photos from Andy hanging in a resident's room. Andy has given me so many pictures that I have started a photo album. These pictures are a valuable reminder of many special times that God has allowed my wife and me to share with our dear friends.

Excerpt from God Cares News

Tips on picture taking:

Some homes are very open and willing to support a ministry such as Andy's, but some are not. New federal privacy laws that went into effect in April 2003 would require that, at the very least, you ask permission of every resident you take a picture of; this may extend even to residents in a group situation. In some cases, someone else (for example, a power of attorney) must grant permission. Some homes may also require written permission. Err on the side of caution and ask first; usually the Director of Activities is the person who will know the nursing home's policy. Remember that pictures or last names of people should never be used without their permission, for example, in a newsletter.

RECEIVING AND GIVING GIFTS IN THE NURSING HOME

On a number of occasions, nursing-home volunteers have asked us, "What do you do when residents try to give you money or other gifts? Should you refuse it, or take it and give it to your church"?

Sometimes a nursing-home resident will feel compelled to give a few dollars or a personal article to a volunteer who ministers at his home. We have been offered money, clothes, food and even a video camera. It is a somewhat awkward situation; we certainly do not visit and minister with the hope of financial or material gain. However, giving is a Biblical responsibility for all Christians; and a resident who wants to give to the Lord's work should be free to obey Him.

Jesus taught that it is more blessed to give than to receive **(Acts 20:35)**. Some of us have learned throughout life that this is true, and so have made giving a way of life. When one of our friends decides to give an offering, we first try to make it clear to him that it is not necessary for him to give to us, that we do not require money or other donations. If he persists in his desire to give, then we receive the donation with gratitude. If this happens more than once or if the valued amount exceeds a few dollars, it is important to inform the director of activities or, if you know the family, you may want to inform them. Explain your position and offer the following:

- To give the money or item back to the family if they are opposed to the giving.
- To offer to use 100% of the funds to cover costs of materials, equipment, etc., for the nursing-home ministry.

It is always best to have certain goals in mind. For this particular situation a good goal is found in ***Romans 14:19: "Let*** *us therefore make every effort to do what leads to peace and mutual edification."*

Tips on giving gifts:

- It is wise to seek permission from the staff before giving gifts; especially any gifts that are breakable, electrical or of high value.
- Writing your friend's name on the article, using permanent marker may help keep it from being lost or stolen.
- Some residents have certain food restrictions or food allergies. Ask permission of the staff before giving any type of food to a resident. Remember, too, that visitors are usually not allowed to feed residents, because of safety concerns.
- Be sensitive when giving gifts that other surrounding residents do not feel left out.

STAFF RELATIONS

As you seek to bless the residents in this mission field, remember there are also many nursing-home staff members who need God's love and Word. Because of their normally very busy schedule, your ministry to them is mostly by example. As they see your faithfulness and genuine love for residents, they will come to appreciate you and may perhaps seek your help to know Christ. Indeed, positive relations with staff can have many worthwhile benefits on the entire nursing-home community.

Occasionally, you might find yourself in quiet conflict with staff members who do not understand or appreciate what the Lord is doing through your ministry. If a conflict arises, Christians need to be the first to examine themselves, pray and respectfully seek a peaceful resolution by talking privately to those involved. Most issues can be worked out through good communication and apologies when mistakes have been made.

However, a few proactive things can be done to nurture good relationships with the staff, as the following example illustrates:

> *It is important to establish positive relationships with the nursing-home staff. Aside from common courtesy and respect, Barry and Linda have taken extra steps to be a blessing to the staff. A few times a year they try to give each staff person a small gift. The gifts are simple; like chocolates to share at the nurse's station, thank-you cards, cookies, prayer cards or even flowers. "It's a small effort that I learned from my dad that really expresses our appreciation of their hard work," said Linda.*
>
> *Sounds like more work? Yes it is. But these seeds of kindness and appreciation often reap good fruit. Some of the noted blessings Barry and Linda have noticed:*

- They receive support, smiles and words of kindness from the staff.
- The residents are being encouraged to go to church.
- Extra effort is made to have the residents up and ready at 9:30 for Sunday morning church.
- Barry and Linda normally have 50 of the 110 residents attend their services. That's about 45% participation. The normal average of group-ministry participation is 15-30%.
- Many of the staff are open to the gospel.

> *Barry notes that many of the people who work on Sunday morning do not attend any church. The only exposure they have with a church is through the care teams that come to the nursing home. We must do what we can, so that they too might know Jesus.*
>
> *God Cares News*

> *If it is possible, as far as it depends on you, live at peace with everyone.*
>
> **Romans 12:18**

There are rare occasions when we do all we can do and still have problems. The following article has been adapted from the Sonshine Society's newsletter:

Staff and management of the nursing home have much to do with creating a welcome atmosphere for the Christian volunteer. It is very important that we as volunteers recognize that they are in a position of authority, and we as volunteers are to be submissive to them and to follow the "rules of the road" in our conduct.

Speaking personally, I have been impressed through the years with the high level of dedication and compassion demonstrated by the personnel I have had opportunity to observe. This is not to say that we see perfection in all staff and management, but is it also... possible?... certain?... that we also are observed to be less than perfect by them?

Like changing tides on the shore, circumstances and staff change in a care center. Some times are better than other times, and some staff are more cooperative than other staff, but our mission remains constant. There is no doubt that it is easier and more rewarding to be received graciously and with open arms by staff and management than to encounter indifference and/or downright antagonism from those in authority. Please remember that should this be the case... it is very likely that the residents still have need of spiritual food and drink, and perhaps even a greater need than those in a friendly environment. We must exercise humility, patience and love. **Only once** *in our 26 years in care-*

center ministry have we encountered outright hostility from staff. Things were done to make our presence very difficult. This finally reached a point where we had to take it to our BOSS. A short time later HE corrected the situation.

Yes, prayer does change things. There have been other little things to endure through the years, but they disappear in the joy of serving our Lord in this area. We would encourage any of you who have experienced or are experiencing less than enthusiastic staff reception, to "hang in there," the tide will turn.

Herm Haakenson, Bits of Sonshine

OTHER SPECIAL CONCERNS

Those who have visitors already:

Occasionally, when you go to visit an individual, someone else will already be there visiting. Normally, you should give way to such prior visitors, although you may wish to get acquainted and talk with them if they seem open to conversation. You should be especially eager to meet your friend's family members. As the occasion arises, introduce yourself, keeping in mind that there may be needs in the family to which the Lord may enable you to respond.

Those who are blind or have limited vision:

Approach the blind person directly and speak to him face to face. Don't assume that because he has difficulty seeing, he also cannot hear. Don't shout; use a normal speaking voice but speak clearly, slowly and distinctly. Touch can be important to a blind person, but speak before you touch him or you may startle him.

Remember the importance of other senses to a blind person, such as smell and touch. For example, if you are bringing a bouquet of flowers, let him smell and touch them. Describe for him things from the environment and your own experience.

Those who are deaf or hard of hearing:

If the person you visit is totally deaf, consider writing or signing as alternatives to verbal communication. It is usually best with the totally deaf to stand facing them so they can see your facial expressions and read your lips. Touching the person gently is a good way of attracting his attention to you before you begin speaking.

If a person is hard of hearing, find out which ear is the "good" ear. Sometimes you may have to speak directly into his ear, but normally standing or sitting on the good side is sufficient. Does he have a hearing aid? Is it turned on? Are the batteries working?

When you speak, speak slowly, distinctly, simply, and at a slow-to-moderate rate of speed. Lower resonance communicates better than greater volume. If you must speak more loudly than normal, be aware that your voice carries and take into account others within earshot. Touch is also important for the hard of hearing

Those who are very sick:

People who are seriously ill are most likely to be bed-bound. They, too, appreciate and need visits. However, do not overtax them; check with the nurses on their condition. Do not stay too long, or demand participation on their part. They may be too weak or in too much pain to communicate verbally. Be alert to eye communication. A gentle touch and few words may be the best expression of love. Words of comfort and assurance and a brief prayer are often quite appropriate.

Those who shout:

Try to decide what the reason for the shouting is. The person may be deaf, hard of hearing, or in need of attention of either a medical or personal sort. There may be a legitimate need that is being ignored. He may have genuine spiritual problems related to unresolved grief or loneliness, for example, and could be "crying for help." On the other hand, this person may be a bit selfish or self-centered. It may be best to speak directly to him about this. Respond appropriately based on your own understanding of the situation. Your unhurried gentle touch along with timely prayer and consoling Scriptures will often be of great comfort.

Those who do not speak English:

Not all residents of care centers will have English as their primary language. If possible, you should arrange for someone who does speak their language to visit them. If you do visit, speak in very simple English. Familiar passages of Scripture or hymns may be helpful in establishing communication. Printed literature can also be useful since some people who cannot speak or understand spoken English can read some English words. Bibles and other religious literature are also available in other languages. (See our Resource Chapter).

Those who are verbally unresponsive:

Sharing your faith with someone who is verbally unresponsive can be a challenge, but it is possible, as the following illustration indicates.

> *Several years ago a couple gave me (Bill) a little 3x5 spiral-bound note pad in which they had written out the plan of salvation in large print. They used this to speak to people who were hearing impaired. A few weeks later, while at a nursing home, I was asked to visit Jerry, who was believed to be near death. When I knelt down next to his bed to talk to him, Jerry looked toward me, but it seemed as if he was looking through me. I was not sure if he could hear me or if he even realized I was there.*
>
> *By faith, I pulled out my little salvation booklet and began to read aloud and put within Jerry's view each page. He showed no emotional*

change or apparent comprehension, but I persevered. As I was finishing up the last page, I asked Jerry to squeeze my hand if he prayed to receive Jesus. I was feeling kind of foolish about having this very one-sided conversation. Suddenly, Jerry spoke, but not with words and tongue but with a smile. I looked over and Jerry gave an ear-to-ear-beaming smile! I stayed with him for a few more minutes as he continued to smile. What a joyful visit!

Jerry continued to live in this nursing home and occasionally was wheeled out to our Bible study. Every time I would see him I would take his hand and say "God bless you, Jerry." Usually he just stared, but sometimes he would give a little smile. One day after greeting Jerry, I expected the usual nonverbal reply, but to my surprise Jerry smiled and also very quietly said "God-----bless -----you." What a joy to know my friend was receiving the many seeds of love.

WHAT IF YOU SEE NEGLECT OR ABUSE?

Neglect

Over the past 19 years of nursing home ministry, I (Bill) have often seen neglect in nursing homes. By neglect, I mean, a lack of willingness or ability of staff members to respond in a timely fashion to a resident's need. There are two sides to neglect. One side is related to the inability of the staff to meet the needs of the residents. It is common for a care center to be understaffed and the caregivers stretched beyond their ability to keep up with all the demands presented. Also, a resident may use his call light several times each hour because he is confused, afraid, lonely or just plain over-demanding. They want anyone to come, and will sometimes make excuses for desired help. Therefore, an unhurried response from the nursing staff could be the reaction of staff members unable to meet requests or inappropriate demands of a resident.

The other side of this issue is willful neglect resulting from laziness, resentment, communication breakdowns and the like.

How do we know the difference? What should we do when we see neglect? The following is a list of questions to consider before you respond to neglect:

- Am I really seeing a true picture of what is happening? There are always two sides to a situation.
- Is this an ongoing situation or an isolated case?
- Is the resident being reasonable in his requests?
- Is the neglect due to an individual worker or is it the overall nursing home or staff issue?
- Is there anything I can do to help?
- Provide a link of respectful communication between the resident and the staff. (Sometimes, merely explaining to the resident that there are almost 100 other residents that the staff is assisting can help him understand and be more accepting of delays.)
- Meet a basic need that a visitor is permitted to do, such as spending time with the resident, praying, building a caring friendship, etc. Becoming his friend and helping him to make friends with his roommate, among his neighbors or in the lounges will enable him to build friendships.

> *If you respectfully inform staff of a resident's needs, your input will be received much better than if you simply tell staff what to do. When approaching staff, it is better to say, "Mrs. Jones has requested help in... I told her that I would inform you," rather than, "Mrs. Jones needs..."*

It is not uncommon to see neglect in a care center. Neglect is not only the care center's staff problem. It is also a family and church problem, as we too become guilty of being too busy or even unwilling to go the extra needed mile to give a drink of water in Jesus' name.

Most regions have Ombudsmen to help mediate between the nursing home and the residents or family members. You can find their phone number in the yellow pages or through your state/province agency for aging. Before calling the Ombudsman, we suggest **first** contacting the facility administration to give them an opportunity to handle the concern.

> *Sometimes staff copes with the ongoing neediness and excessive call light use by getting sort of "used" to it. It doesn't make it right, it just is a way that they can cope with the work load and the emotional load of working with all those dependent people. Some employees that are new to this kind of work think that anyone can do this job, and then find out how demanding it is. Turnover and call-offs, especially within the first 90 days is probably over 75% in most homes. Also, some of the people that take caregiver jobs have limited emotional resources for handling their own stresses. Its tough to be kicked, called names, spit at by elderly residents* **That doesn't mean it's OK to retaliate,** *but it gets very challenging for staff with limited coping skills.*
>
> *A Director of Nursing*

Abuse

Abuse is an issue that is much more severe than neglect. While neglect is often due to busyness or unwillingness to respond in a timely fashion to a person's needs, abuse is the act of purposefully harming or taking advantage of a person. Abuse could include:

- Physical: hitting, pinching, shoving or pushing; handling roughly or administering a treatment roughly.
- Verbal: yelling, insulting, demeaning; threats or comments that result in emotional damage or amount to mental cruelty.
- Sexual molestation
- Financial: theft or scamming
- Prolonged neglect, such as leaving a person in soiled linen.

Such activity is extremely inappropriate and must be reported to the proper authorities. If you ever see abuse in a care center, we recommend the following response.

- Try to stop any actual ongoing act by letting your presence be seen.
- Write down any details, i.e., time, location, people involved, words said, etc.
- Report incident to the unit manager. If he is not available, report to the director of nurses or administrator.

It is best to let the management handle the issue. There are specific procedures that they are required, by law, to follow when abuse is reported. They are required to do an extensive investigation and suspend anyone that has been accused until the investigation is complete. Action may involve terminating the abuser's employment and even criminal prosecution.

In some rare instances, the nursing-home management may not respond appropriately to your report. Another option is to contact the State Elder Abuse Hotline. We highly recommend that this is done **only** after you have tried the above procedures and have not seen appropriate response from the management. Calling the state in, can at times, create more trouble for the management than what they deserve. Although abuse is entirely unacceptable, try to work with the staff for a satisfactory resolution.

> **Do not be overcome by evil, but overcome evil with good.**
>
> **Romans 12:21**

Reporting abuse may be a risk to the witness, as the abuser may seek revenge. We recommend that you be careful to protect yourself from this concern by: not openly talking to others about the event and asking authorities to keep your name concealed as much as possible.

Remember also that the abuser may be reacting to a deeper personal problem that they need help with. Although personal problems do not excuse abusive behavior and the need for accountability, ministering to the abuser may be the best form of future prevention.

The most effective defense against neglect and abuse is the presence of caring family and friends. Constant visits at random times from a caring family member or friend will do more to protect and support a nursing-home resident than any rule or government regulation. Some of these points are also made by a director of nurses:

> *The very best thing that the residents can have to protect them from abuse and/or neglect is frequent involved visitors. It's the same reason that when you go into a store, the clerks make eye contact and greet you--it stops misconduct in stores. So if family/friends are in and out of the facility, everyone knows that you have to answer for that resident's care to someone who cares about them.*

"Acts of love are works of peace." Mother Teresa

CHAPTER 12

MINISTERING TO THE GRIEVING AND THE DYING

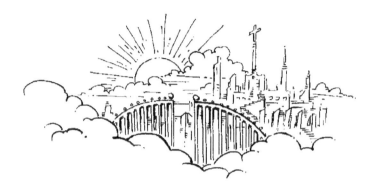

On one occasion at the nursing home, a nurse informed me (Bill) that a resident, whom I will call Maxine, asked to see me. I had seen Maxine in the lounge but never had the chance to sit with her before this time. It was during this first visit that she expressed a desire to make peace with God. She was very sincere and open about her past sins. I did not have to convince her of her need for Jesus, I only had to explain for her the way to Him. She was able to read, so after we prayed, I gave her a large print Gospel of John.

Later that day I saw a nurse who expressed gratitude for my willingness to spend time with Maxine. I thought how fortunate "I" was to have shared with her. The following week I returned to visit Maxine. She asked for more reading material and I gave her a New Testament. I visited for a few more weeks, and then, less frequently because she would usually be sleeping when I stopped by.

Then one day I received a message from the family calling me to her bedside as Maxine was just hours away from passing on. Her family, who did not attend church, told me how Maxine had spoken so highly of me and they asked me if I would pray for her. What a privilege! Later I was asked to share at her memorial service, which I did. I shared with her family my hope that because of Maxine's trust in Jesus she was now with Him in heaven. I also shared that this was possible for anyone else who accepted Jesus as his or her Savior. After the service I had no contact with the family except for a thank-you card. My wife and I had only hoped and prayed that God's Word had reached good soil.

Three years went by and one day I received a call from Maxine's oldest daughter asking if I would speak at the funeral for her sister, who had just died in an auto accident. She explained how her sister, who was an alcoholic, was touched by the message I had shared at her mother's memorial service. The funeral had been the event that was the beginning of her sister's seeking to change her life, turning from alcohol to Jesus. Because of this, the whole family asked for me to conduct the funeral service. Again, I shared the Word of God with the hope of watering some previously planted seeds. This time we did see evidence of hearts being touched.

As missionaries to people in nursing homes, we will have opportunities to visit and minister to residents who are dying. We will also encounter many people who have lost friends and loved ones and are having difficulty coping with doubts, fears and the sorrows that can accompany their loss. Through the guidance of the Holy Spirit, our visits can bring great comfort and hope as we point our friends to the Lord Jesus Christ, their Savior and Comforter.

This chapter is written to provide some helpful suggestions for comforting nursing-home residents, family members, nursing-home staff, and even yourself. In addition to the material in this chapter, we recommend you search out other resources that can help you better understand grief and death from a Biblical perspective.

GRIEF DEFINED

Grief can be defined as emotional suffering; it generally includes periods of deep sorrow. We often associate grief with death, but there are many other causes usually associated in some way with loss. Examples include the loss of a relationship through divorce, or a significant role change, as when a spouse becomes the caregiver to his life partner. Grief can also be triggered by the loss of health, the loss of a job, the death of a pet, or even relocation to another community. Sometimes, seemingly small issues are a major source of grief for another person, for example, the loss of treasured possessions that can occur when a person must relocate to a nursing home where there is no room for such items.

Grief can be expressed in many ways: shock, crying, anger, guilt, panic, loss of appetite, overwhelming fatigue, bitterness, depression, loneliness and extreme and fluctuating emotions. Many authors have identified different stages of grief to help us better understand its nature and even its benefits. It is important to realize, however, that many people may go back and forth among various stages. There is no set pattern or amount of time for people to advance through grief. Even when one can settle into a final stage of acceptance, the reality and sense of loss still remains, requiring ongoing adjustments.

The best gift one can offer to someone who is grieving is a listening ear. Words should generally be used sparingly, and the most comforting words can be as simple as "I'm sorry" or "I care." A hug, a hand on a shoulder, shared tears, a squeeze of the hand and the offer to pray with or for a person will communicate that you care, and can be a great kindness to the person who is grieving.

THERE IS A GOOD AND GODLY GRIEF

Although grief can be the result of a number of different kinds of losses or major changes, here, we will focus primarily on ministering to people who are grieving because of the death of a loved one. You will find that the principles for helping a grieving friend are very similar for most sources for grief.

The death of a loved one is one of the most challenging events that one can face in life. There are many different feelings and emotions that people can experience when facing the loss of a beloved friend or a family member. The following factors can significantly impact the grieving process in either positive or negative ways:

- The grieving person's understanding of and relationship with God.
- The departed person's relationship or lack of relationship with God, especially if the grieving person has a strong faith.
- How long and well the grieving person knew the departed person.
- How much the grieving person depended on the departed person.

- The quality of the relationship between the grieving and the departed person.

We have the ability to do much good for the nursing-home resident, for family members and for staff through our compassionate words, attitudes and actions. We must also be sensitive during times of others' grieving, to not speak in haste as certain words can do harm.

Reckless words pierce like a sword, but the tongue of the wise brings healing (Proverbs 12:18).

Everyone grieves following the loss of a loved one, but not all people grieve in the same way. Some people react immediately with great sorrow. Some have a delayed reaction. Some appear to recover in a relatively short time. For others, the grieving process may take many years before the person feels he can actually move on in his own life. Grief is not only common, it is also healthy, if handled properly. We must be careful not to try to put a stop to a person's mourning or grief. Christians can sometimes be guilty of this by attributing a lengthy period of grieving or mourning to a lack of faith. The verse that is sometimes used to justify this attitude is **I Thessalonians 4:13** when Paul says: *"Brothers, we do not want you to be ignorant about those who fall asleep, or to grieve like the rest of men, who have no hope."* As believers, we know that the death of a believing loved one is only a temporary separation. We know that in our Father's time, we will all share eternity together in joyful assembly. People who do not understand or believe in God's plan for His children lack such hope and are subject to intense despair. Our hope gives us the grace to take Jesus' hand and to press on in His promises. Yet, this hope does not prevent the experience of grief during our personal loss; especially at the loss of close relatives like a child or a spouse.

In the Bible, we find that people mourned for several days at the death of loved ones. In **Acts 8:2** we read that *"Godly men buried Stephen and mourned deeply for him."* In **Genesis 49 & 50** Joseph mourned for Jacob 70 days. Israel mourned for Moses 30 days. Paul almost lost a good friend, but his friend was finally healed, sparing Paul *"sorrow upon sorrow"(Philippians 2:27).*

The grieving or potential grieving these people experienced was not because there was no hope of eternity; they were simply experiencing profound personal loss that is part of our shared humanity.

Jesus also experienced and understood grief. In *Isaiah 53:2-3* we read this prophetic passage: *He has no form or comeliness; And when we see Him, There is no beauty that we should desire Him. He is despised and rejected by men, A Man of sorrows and acquainted with grief. And we hid, as it were, our faces from Him; He was despised, and we did not esteem Him.* (NKJV) When Jesus wept at the tomb of His friend Lazarus, no one said to Him, "Don't worry, have faith in God, he will rise again." It says in *John 11:33-36, "He was deeply moved in spirit and troubled.. ...Jesus wept. Then the Jews said, 'See how he loved him!'"*

> *My experience (Bill) through the death of close friends and family, is that they leave voids in my heart and mind. No one or nothing can replace them; but, in time, the Lord sends new friends into my life to fill some of these voids. As I reach out in Christ's love to others, I find that God uses me to lessen the grief of others as well.*

HOW CAN I HELP?

Grief is a journey that is unique for each person. Throughout the journey, one needs to learn to see things from God's perspective; in doing so, a person can find peace, hope, and the courage to move on. The key element for a successful journey is a continual increasing faith in the Lord Jesus Christ.

We can help people along their grief journey by remembering the following points:

- Be a friend. Learn to sincerely listen and pray, give a warm and gentle hug when appropriate, and communicate caring by words and actions.

- Do not be afraid to reminisce with the person about their departed loved one or ask positive questions about them; this often helps people to release bound-up emotions and to sort out confusing thoughts. Often people want to talk about the lost one, but other people do not enable them, fearing this might be upsetting. Sometimes people enjoy looking at old photos of their loved one and would appreciate sharing their memories with someone who will simply listen but is not as emotionally invested.

- Walk with them through the grief process (even literally taking a walk can help!), but do not try to lead a person out of grief; let him move at his own pace. Grief is not a problem to be fixed, but a journey to be embarked upon, preferably with caring friends. Take the advice Paul gives the believers in Rome and *Mourn with those who mourn (Romans 12:15).*

- Encourage and help a grieving person walk closer to Jesus through prayer, Scripture reading, Christian fellowship, and even, when appropriate, encouraging him to reach out to someone else who is mourning. Do your best and leave the rest up to the Lord.

My comfort in my suffering is this: Your promise preserves my life (Psalm 119:50).

Understanding the grief journey will also prevent us from saying words that cause more harm than good. The following phrases are expressions that are generally **unhelpful** and should be avoided:

- You shouldn't feel like that.

- I know how you feel.
- You should be getting over it by now.
- It could have been worse.
- It must be God's will.
- You're not the only one to have experienced this.
- Don't cry; everyone is looking up to you.
- Call me if you need me. (It is better for you to call to see if there is a need.)
- We'll have you over some time. (It is better, when you are able and prepared, to call and invite, or just show up at their door with a willingness to share your time.)

Such comments usually hurt rather than help those who are grieving. They are often used when a helper is uncomfortable with grief or trying to stop the process. Sincere words like: "I am sorry; that must have been difficult for you," can be sensitive and meaningful. Keep in mind, however, that there are times, (especially during anger) that there are not any correct words to say. Fervent prayer, seeking the help of mature believers and treating others the way you would want to be treated will always bear good fruit.

MINISTERING TO THE DYING

To die in peace with God is the culmination of any human life.

Of those who have died in our houses, I have never seen anyone die in despair or cursing. They have all died serenely.

I took a man I had picked up from the street to our Home for the Dying in Calcutta. When I was leaving, he told me, "I have lived like an animal on the streets, but I am going to die like an angel. I will die smiling."

He did die smiling, because he felt loved and surrounded by care. That is the greatness of our poor!

Mother Teresa, *In My Own Words*

~~~ * ~~~

When I go to the bedside of one who is dying, I speak only words of comfort and peace. I believe Jesus is merciful to the suffering elderly. I tell them to take the hand of Jesus and that He will lead them home to a place of comfort, light and peace. I tell them they will soon be strong and beautiful. I tell them it will be a joyful assembly and soon we will all be there, too!

Sometimes, if I don't know the person, I will pray a prayer of inviting Jesus into their heart or life. I say the words for them and ask them to agree. I know that God is merciful – His mercy endures forever.

<div align="right">Mary Ann Goodrich</div>

Sometimes you may be given the privilege to minister to a person who is near death. As with all aspects of nursing-home ministry, there is not one set pattern that should be used in all situations. There are, however, a few principles to remember that can help you bring hope and comfort to the person facing death.

Try to assess their situation:

Is he afraid of death or at peace? Is his fear or peace based on truth? Is any hope based in a personal relationship with Jesus Christ or in personal righteousness? Some people may have fears about death because they do not believe in Jesus. Others who do not believe in Jesus may appear to have no fear.

Respectfully share the Word of God:

You can encourage your friend to read passages that focus on salvation, heaven, and the transition of dying; they may hear directly from God as they read such Scriptures. If they are unable to read, read it for them slowly, giving time for them to reflect on the words and on any areas of concern. One helpful passage of Scripture is ***John 14:6: Jesus said, "I am the way and the truth and the life. No man comes to the Father but through me."*** In this same chapter, Jesus speaks about going to heaven to prepare a place for the believer. This passage can be of great comfort, as Jesus also promises to come again and walk with them through the valley or process of death, ushering them into the presence of God, their Father. **Psalm 23** is also one of the most comforting Psalms for a believer. **John 3, Romans 8** and **1 Corinthians 15** also have many helpful verses to share. We must be careful to speak to this person from the perspective of a friend, not as a judge or counselor. We do well to see ourselves as helpers for those who are seekers. Singing hymns and spiritual songs may also be a great encouragement.

Speak with hope and faith:

Many people who are very near death are not able to talk much. They are usually struggling to breathe and may seem as if they do not know what is happening around them. Their appearance should not prevent you from ministering to them. If your friend is verbally unresponsive, you can ask him to squeeze your hand to affirm that he hears you. Even if the person cannot respond or squeeze your hand, it is still quite possible that he can hear and understand your words. Still, when someone is unable to understand your words, he most often can feel your loving presence. Share with him, in faith, that the Lord will enable him to hear and understand your words.

Be patient:

Speaking (or singing) words of hope, in an unhurried compassionate spirit, will normally bring peace. If your friend seems to be agitated when you talk about the Lord or bring up the subject of dying, you can reminisce with him by talking about pictures or articles in the room, or past experiences that you may know about. Sharing encouraging past memories may take your friend's mind off the immediate fears and ease the tension. Then, gradually turning to the promises of the Lord and prayer may allow for a more receptive response.

What you might say when in doubt:

If you are unclear about the dying person's faith and relationship with Jesus Christ you might say the following:

"I am concerned that you will be departing soon. One of the biggest concerns I have when people are facing their last days on earth is whether they are prepared to meet the Lord Jesus. I wish we were able to talk about it but since you cannot speak, I thought I would read a few Scriptures and pray for you."

You can then read examples of those who called upon the Lord Jesus, repented of sins, and make peace with Him.

Always consider – what would I want someone to do for me if I were dying? How would I want a friend to walk with me and talk to me? The Lord will guide you as you prayerfully seek to bless your friend.

Helpful Scriptures to use with a person facing death include: **Psalms 23, 25, 51, 90, 103, John 14** and **Romans 8**. It is very helpful to have in your possession a pocketsize New Testament (NT) with Psalms, with these and other meaningful verses highlighted. Be familiar with them and remember you do not have to read every verse within the chapter, just what is beneficial for your friend. See also **Ephesians 4:29** and **2 Timothy 2:15.** Sharing Scripture which have been personally meaningful to you in times of grief and loss can also be helpful for a dying person.

If family is present:

If you arrive in the room and the family is present, respectfully introduce yourself and discern if you are welcome at this time. Avoid talking to the family while ignoring the resident, or talking about the resident with family in front of the resident. As soon as you sense you're welcome, begin to talk to the resident. Tell him that it is nice to see his family at his side. Affirm their concern for him. Read the Scriptures and sing some hymns; take your time in seeking to bring comfort to the resident and family. Before you leave, invite all present to hold hands as you lead a prayer for their loved one, if they are comfortable with that. Do not use your prayer as an opportunity to preach. Let your prayer be a prayer of comfort and support. Just talk to the Lord and ask Him to give mercy and comfort by His grace.

> *Norma was a resident of the nursing home we visit, and she was close to death. We had been friends for a couple of years and I (Bill) knew she trusted and loved Jesus. However, her husband, Earl, whom I had met a few times before, did not show any signs of faith in Christ. When the time came for Norma's departure from this world, Earl and I stood at her bedside. I struggled for words because I knew Norma was fine and would be in the future, but Earl was grieving without hope. After making a few comments, Earl looked at me and said, "You haven't done this much, have you?" I said, "No, I am sorry, I haven't; I just don't know what to say except that I have hope that she is OK because she loves and trusts Jesus".*
>
> *At the time, I felt like I had failed Earl; that my words were in vain. A few years later while walking down the hall of the same nursing home, I glanced into a room and there in a wheelchair was Earl. We had a very warm exchange of words*

and reminisced about Norma. Through his affirming words, I realized at that time that God's grace was sufficient in my weakness.

FUNERAL OR MEMORIAL SERVICES

The funeral service is distinguished from the memorial service chiefly by the relationship of the body of the deceased to the worship service. In a funeral service, the body is either present or is an integral part of the funeral process. But the body is neither present for, nor a part of, the memorial service. The word "funeral" comes from a Sanskrit work meaning "smoke," and refers to the rites used in the disposition of a dead human body. The worship service may properly be called a funeral service if the body is laid to rest immediately prior to or after the service, although not present in the service. A memorial service or services may be held at the same time as the funeral service, or at other times, or on the anniversary of a death.
From Abingdon Funeral Manual, 1976, pp 18-21

As your relationship with residents and their family members grows closer, you may be asked to conduct a funeral or memorial service. This honor and privilege is normally given to ordained ministers and it is appropriate to ask the family if the deceased person is affiliated with a church; if this is the case, you might encourage them to first consider that their pastor conduct the service with you assisting him. There may be legitimate reasons, however, for the family not to have the pastor of a church conduct the service, but it is common courtesy to ask. In most states it is not a requirement for the officiator of a funeral service be an ordained minister, but their support will be a great asset.

Funerals are an opportunity to invest into the lives of many people, especially relatives and close friends of nursing-home residents. Although you are encouraged to share the gospel in your service, please remember your primary function is to be a source of comfort through hope and the Word of God. If your primary goal is to preach a salvation message, you may fall short of bringing comfort. However, if your primary goal is to comfort the mourners with hope and the Word of God, the Gospel will naturally be part of your message. A truly successful funeral service helps the attendees embrace the hope that Jesus offers. This hope will help carry them through the grieving process.

Preparing for the Service

You can lead a service that is both meaningful and life-giving to the family and friends. There are funeral manuals and service guidebooks for ministers that provide detailed outlines, guidelines and Scripture references that can help you understand various denominational traditions and what some people may prefer in a service. We recommend that you do not use this resource alone. Prayer, family input, and support from your pastor are all important resources. If you have reasonable assurance that the person is now in heaven, an alternative name for a funeral service can be a *homecoming celebration.*

If the family asks you to conduct a service outside of the nursing home, you should meet with them to plan and establish the dimensions of the service according to their needs and desires. The funeral home will work out the service time and location, but the family will need you to take the lead on how the actual services will be conducted. Your meeting should take place as soon as most of the close family members are available. Your warm, understanding presence and honesty will bring much comfort to this gathering. You will need to be prepared to take notes as you learn as much about the person as possible. Start out by asking for common information such as would be shared in the obituary. Then ask about achievements or significant events that took place in his life. This may lead into a great time of reminiscing, giving much comfort.

You may want to let the family know that the service is for the family and friends and it does not have to be in keeping with normal traditions. Encourage them to make a collage on poster board or encourage some other way of displaying pictures. This is very meaningful and will help to break tension during calling hours or the funeral itself. Ask if the departed loved one had any favorite Scriptures, hymns, poems, or songs that could be included in the service; these will also tell you a lot about the person's faith. Ask if family or friends would like to say anything during the service. Be prepared to answer if they ask you how much you charge for the service. A very important part of this gathering will be to close with prayer; hands can be held if appropriate. This may be the first and only time a family has ever shared in prayer together. If troublesome issues are brought up, such as unresolved conflicts with the deceased, practice your listening skills and offer encouragement and guidance for forgiveness; it may also be very helpful to include some thoughts on forgiveness in the actual message. Closing in prayer, asking the Lord to intervene, will likely be the greatest help, as He will bring peace to the humble-hearted. Be sensitive and try not to preach as you pray. It normally does not happen, but if issues arise for which you cannot provide appropriate support, you can encourage professional help or offer your own church's intervention. Finally, as time permits, we recommend that you go to the viewing services to be available for additional support and comfort.

It is very important to prepare a personalized service and be involved with the family as much as they seem to need you. Following are some guidelines and tips for conducting a funeral service, usually conducted outside of the nursing home; and for memorial services, usually conducted inside the nursing home. Often other nursing-home residents will want to be present in the nursing-home memorial services, though this would be based on the family's wishes.

A recommended format for a funeral service:

- Arrive at the service location early, spiritually prepared and with fresh breath.
- Opening hymn and/or Scripture.
- Invocation - (opening prayer to ask for God's blessing).
- Introduction with biographical summary – Example: We are gathered here today in memory of our friend John R. Doe who died (or, if a known Christian, who has gone to be with Jesus) on Thursday, October 12, 2022. John was born… in the town of… He was the husband of.., the father of.., etc. (This information comes from the family meeting and the funeral home.)
- Welcome- Express appreciation for all those who have taken the time to come to be with the family and friends.
- Scripture- The following are some helpful Scriptures passages that could be read during the service; some passages may need to be shortened to suit your needs. Be selective. Family members may also desire to be involved in the selection of Scripture.
  - Psalm 23, 39, 46, 90, 103, 121, 130
  - Matthew 11:28-30
  - John 5:24-29, 11: 25-26, 14:1-6 & 25-28, 16:33
  - Romans 8:16-17 & 28 & 31-39
  - 1 Corinthians 15
  - 2 Corinthians 4:17, 5:5
  - Revelation 7:9-17, 21:1-4, 22:3-5
- Testimonies- Reflections from family or friends. Do not limit their time - within reason.
- If you knew the deceased, share your own testimony/reflections. (This adds a personal touch that is appreciated by all.)
- Meditation – The meditation is Scriptural sharing, normally less than ten minutes long with a primary focus

on the promises and faithfulness of Jesus. The primary thrust should not be evangelism, but feel free to explain the way to Jesus, using perhaps, **John 14**, and the joy and security of knowing Him. It should be a blessing to the family and friends and provide lots of hope.

- A hymn related to the meditation.
- Closing prayer.
- The Funeral Director will make necessary announcements.
- If there is a graveside service, try to be present, walking in front of the casket while the pallbearers are moving it.

The graveside service is normally very short, but it is often a very important time for the family as a final process of letting go.

A recommended format for a graveside service:

- Be at the hearse when the casket is removed. Lead the way to the gravesite without getting in the way.
- Share a very short devotional to remind the people of God's promises.
- A prayer of releasing the person into the hands of the Merciful Savior.
- A closing prayer and final benediction. - Go in the peace and hope of our LORD Jesus Christ.
- The Funeral Director will make necessary announcements.
- Do not be in a hurry to leave. Your presence is most often appreciated.
- Try to go to the after-service gathering. This is sometimes the best time for further ministry.

The nursing-home staff may approach you, or you may want to approach them, to conduct an in-home memorial service or service of remembrance for the staff and residents. Homes often conduct memorial services annually or quarterly to honor and remember residents who have died. The above format could be modified or followed for both types of services.

Here is another suggested format that can be adapted for different situations:

A recommended format for a nursing-home memorial service or a service of remembrance:

- As residents gather for the service, quiet background music should be played. Sometimes a small group plays instrumental music, for example, violins or a harp, if available.

- Welcome those who have come; remind them that this service is a time to remember with hope. You might have one 10-15 minute meditation or several short meditations interspersed with songs and hymns based on different themes, for example, hope, love, joy, peace or forgiveness.

- One very effective type of service incorporates the use of candles, especially if family members or staff are present. A large candle can be lit in the front of the room. At the appropriate time, a family member or staff member can come forward with a candle representing a person who has died and is being remembered, light the candle from the larger candle and place it in a candle holder. Names of the people being remembered are then read. An alternative is the use of cut flowers that can be carried in individually and then placed in a vase or in individual flower holders. (Note when using candles: fire is always a safety hazard; abide by the rules of the nursing home and use caution.)

- If only a few people are being remembered, time can be given for the audience to share memories of one of them.

- It is often a blessing to have pictures of the people being remembered placed on a table in the front of the room.

- After the candle lighting, there might be a time of silent meditation when instrumental music or a quiet hymn is

played. Someone might sing a solo or duet, focusing on the love of God and the hope we have in Christ.
- Close with a congregational hymn and benediction.
- Light refreshments are often served following this type of service so that people can continue to reminisce.

Follow-up

It is a good idea to call the person who asked you to perform the funeral or memorial service, a week, and then a month, after the service, and also in the coming year during a special holiday such as a birthday or anniversary. This call will be to encourage the family and to see if there are any spiritual needs to which you can offer support. Take your time on these phone calls and offer prayer, if appropriate. You may also want to encourage church attendance and Bible reading. Most importantly, just be a friend in Jesus. Keep a record of services you are asked to lead, and a record for follow-up times, so you do not forget. Also remember that when a person dies in a nursing home, there is often a grieving roommate. Even if the two people were not well acquainted, at the very least the surviving roommate may be personally struggling with his own mortality. He might be very appreciative of a follow-up visit.

The Lord can use you to impart peace and hope, sometimes sparing those left behind unnecessary pain and sorrow, even though they will continue to grieve. It can be a great comfort to family and friends to know that others cared about and remembered their loved one.

As we abide in Christ, He sends His heavenly treasures through us, to heal the broken-hearted and bind up their wounds. God will give you the words to speak as you minister to the grieving and the dying. Remember, verse **1** of **Psalm 23** also applies to you: ***The Lord is my shepherd, I shall not want.***

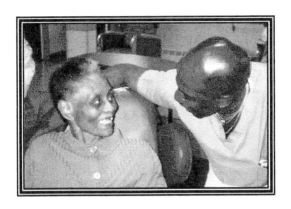

Jesus said, "I tell you the truth, anyone who has faith in me will do what I have been doing. He will do even greater things than these, because I am going to the Father. And I will do whatever you ask in my name, so that the Son may bring glory to the Father" (John 14:12-13).

THE HIDDEN TREASURE

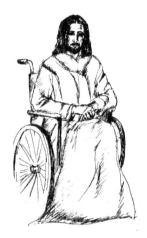

"Come, you who are blessed by my Father; take your inheritance, the kingdom prepared for you since the creation of the world. For I was hungry and you gave me something to eat, I was thirsty and you gave me something to drink, I was a stranger and you invited me in, I needed clothes and you clothed me, I was sick and you looked after me, I was in prison and you came to visit me" (Matthew 25:34-36).

As ambassadors of Christ, we recognize our responsibility to reach out to help people living in nursing homes. However, it seems that there just is not enough time to do all the things there are to do. Therefore, we must choose to leave behind the less important things and lay hold of the better and greater things. Scripture points out how Mary chose what was better, as she took the time away from a busy schedule to be with Jesus (**Luke 10:40-42**).

Have you ever wondered what it must have been like for the disciples to sit at Jesus' feet and listen to the heart of our heavenly Father speaking through Him? It would be easy to drop any activities for the privilege to be near Him. **Matthew 25:40** reminds us that whatever we do for one who is less fortunate, we are actually doing for Jesus. This means that our Lord Jesus is somehow intimately connected with the residents of the nursing homes. As we come to realize this fact, our "duty" to visit becomes a "privilege." Our responsibility to minister is transformed into desire. Instead of giving Him the leftovers of our time and resources, we gladly lavish on Him our first fruits.

What a great privilege our Lord has afforded us: to touch

> "Does it make you a king to have more and more cedar? Did not your father have food and drink? He did what was right and just, so all went well with him. He defended the cause of the poor and needy, and so all went well. Is that not what it means to know me?" declares the LORD.
> **Jeremiah 22:15-16**

Him and love Him in such a tangible way. When we lay hold of the greater duties of life, we will be laying hold of Jesus Himself, and our joy will be full! **(John 15:10-11).**

> *There once was a women whose two-year-old child was dying of a bone disease. The only thing that could save the child's life was a bone-marrow transplant. After much searching, and as the child was very near death, a woman of no importance to her community was discovered to have the right blood match. Soon she was rushed to the hospital where the procedure was immediately performed. The result was that the child lived and became very healthy. Now, who was most grateful, the two-year-old child or the mother? The child would have only a surface understanding of what was happening; whereas the mother would have a much deeper understanding and appreciation for the donor and her sacrifice. What would this loving mother not have given to save her child?*

In the same way, when we help a nursing-home resident escape eternal death or offer any charity to bless them, we are doing it for Jesus. Jesus is so deeply concerned and in love with the weak that He would give us anything we need to help them.

> *Jesus said, "And if anyone gives even a cup of cold water to one of these little ones because he is my disciple, I tell you the truth, he will certainly not lose his reward" (Matthew 10:42).*

~~~~ PRAYER ~~~~

May our Lord Jesus enable us always to discover the great treasures hidden behind every sacrifice given in His love. And may His kingdom come, and His will be done, in every care center; to the glory and honor of our Father.

Jesus said, "Now that you know these things, you will be blessed if you do them" John 13:17.

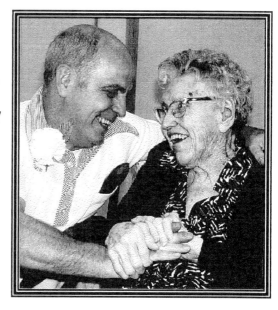

ACKNOWLEDGEMENTS

I (Tom) have had the privilege of getting to know and work with Bill and Mary Ann Goodrich, camping out in their home, praying together, sharing dreams and visions, passions and frustrations. I am very honored to share the writing of this book with Bill, whom the Lord has taught much and used in many, many untold ways both in nursing homes and in the lives of those he has trained and encouraged, myself included. I want to thank them first of all.

There are, however, many other people who are to be thanked for their part along the way. Deserving of special mention would, first of all, be Dr. John Skilton. He is remembered fondly, with admiration and appreciation, and with the abiding prayer that I might be more and more like him, as he exemplified Jesus in so many wonderful ways. For her assistance both in the past and with the current editing and encouragement I thank Sharon Fish Mooney. And for assistance in many personal and practical ways, including promotion and support of the developing of my involvement in Nursing-Home Ministries. I wish to give special mention and appreciation to Marlene Hammerschmidt, Steve, Karen, Dr. Jack Miller and the elders and deacons of New Life Church, Georgina, Penny, and many others who typed, edited, mimeographed, compiled, and distributed versions of training materials and greeting cards. And not a few cups of cold water, hot coffee and kind words were also served along the way. Thanks to each one, each in a special way, the unnamed at least as much as the named. God has used you as a blessing, has blessed you, and surely will continue to do so.

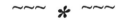

In addition to the many people who have supported Tom, I (Bill), would like to offer my acknowledgements. First, my thanks my thanks go to my wife Mary Ann, whose love and sensitivity for the residents we minister to has always influenced and amazed me.

Tom McCormick, with whom I have enjoyed a rich fellowship for over 10 years that has helped to mold my heart and life. Our partnership in this writing project has been a privilege and a blessing to me. Herm Haakenson, founder and former president of the SonShine Society was my mentor in this mission field and an example to me of Jesus. Herm was full of wisdom, humor and love for all people, especially his family and the residents of care centers. Heaven is filled with saints like Herm. Thanks also to Sharon Fish Mooney, our editor and friend, whose experience, support, skills and sacrifices have made it possible to blend Tom's and my thoughts into what I trust will be a very helpful tool for nursing-home missionaries. Her input into this book has been invaluable. Deep appreciation and thanks to the thousands of nursing-home residents I have been blessed to know and touch since 1984. They have helped me to discover the true treasures of heaven as over and over Christ has made Himself known to me through them. He has used them to teach and bless me beyond words.

There are several others who have shared their time and ideas; they include my friends Marilyn Barrett, Greg Jevnikar, Nicole Fraser, Carol Altman, Fran Palffy, Ruth Dodds, Carolyn Herrmann. Special thanks to my loyal office assistants, Dena Pincombe and Pam Case. I also want to acknowledge and thank my family, who through their support and sacrifices have enabled me to share my life with many others. God bless you all!

Finally, I want to thank our Lord Jesus Christ who reached down very low to save my life and gave me true purpose, hope, peace and treasured friends beyond number.

RESOURCES AND RESOURCE PEOPLE

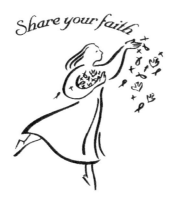

One of the challenges we veteran nursing-home missionaries faced twenty years ago was the lack of ministry resources available for the work. Today, we are much better supplied with large print Scriptures, music resources, cards and devotionals that were designed for this harvest field. We are quite grateful to those who have developed and published these resources as they usually come via sacrifice. We have listed many of these resources as well as books, newsletters and tapes that directly or indirectly provide help for this ministry.

Another great resource available to us is the many nursing-home ministries that have been established to help Christians develop Christ-centered care teams. We begin this chapter with profiles describing a few of these ministries and the resources they provide. We have been very encouraged and blessed to have met and now network with the directors of these other ministries and encourage you to contact the ones near you. Together, the Lord is using all of us to advance His kingdom in every long-term care center. What a privilege we share!

If you are aware of other resources that should be added to this list, feel free to contact us that we may consider it in our next printing.

CHAPTER & VERSE MINISTRIES, INC.

1543 Norcova Ave.
Norfolk, VA 23502-1720
Phone: 757-714-3133
Website: www.chapterandverse.org
Email: chapnvers@chapterandverse.org

The vision of Chapter and Verse Ministries is to spread the Gospel of Jesus Christ and promote unity in the body of Christ.

Their mission: They use three tools in fulfilling their vision: 1.) Small-group Bible study and prayer. 2.) Publication of Christian poetry. 3.) Motivating and empowering Christians to volunteer in their local care facilities.

President and Director of Ministry: Gerald T. Johnson

This work began in the spring of 1991 as an effort to respond to the need for an interdenominational, unified approach to meeting the volunteer needs of Hampton Roads, VA, care facilities.

They present the needs to the Christian community and supply willing volunteers with helpful materials and resources. Chapter & Verse also coordinates with the care-facility staff and trains volunteers as needed. Activities they have coordinated include one-to-one visiting, transportation for residents, chaperones for resident field trips, Christian entertainment, care-package programs and distribution of large-print Scriptures and magazines.

Resources:

- "A Handbook for Nursing Home Ministry". This is a 200 page guide with ideas, tools, and resources for care-facility ministry. (Available in printed format or on their website.)
- Large-print hymnbook with accompaniment CD.

COMMUNITY CHAPLAIN SERVICES
PO Box 6734
New Bedford, MA 02742-6734
Phone & Fax: 508-997-3174
Email: commchap@surfglobal.net

The vision of Community Chaplain Services is to provide Bible-believing chaplains in secular nursing homes. Chaplains provide friendship, comfort and encouragement for Christian residents and encourage a vital faith in Jesus Christ to the lost and lonely.

Their mission as an evangelical faith home mission is to engage and send career and part-time missionary chaplains for ministry in nursing homes, with the two thrusts of evangelism and pastoral care. They also train laymen and women to serve part-time in the nursing homes.

Ministry Director: Walter Dryer

CCS was founded in 1972 by Rev. David Kimball as a church outreach into the secular sector of our society, where the need is great, and so little ministry is found. CCS currently has full-time or part-time (lay) chaplains serving in all the New England states, as well as New York, Pennsylvania, Delaware, Wisconsin, Florida, Arizona and in New Brunswick, Canada. As a faith mission, CCS requires of its chaplains a definite call to this field, raising of modest support through deputation, and CCS training. We invite qualified persons who have had satisfactory careers as pastors and missionaries to serve with CCS as nursing home missionary chaplains.

Resources:
CCS has developed their own materials, which they will gladly share.

DESERT MINISTRIES, INC.
PO Box 4704
Omaha, NE 68104
Phone: 402-556-8032
Fax: 402-551-8581
Website: www.desertministries.org
Email: info@desertministries.org

The vision of Desert Ministries is to develop programs to promote intergenerational contact wherever possible, and educate congregations about the aging process and their responsibilities as Christians to serve the frail elderly.

Their mission is to reach into long-term care facilities to support the people who live there, their families, and the care staff.

For the residents, they recruit and train volunteers to befriend and combat loneliness and depression. For the families, they provide spiritual support through a prayer chain, and practical support by networking them with local support agencies. For the care staff, they present in-services, and workshops to give them the tools to meet the spiritual needs of their patients, their peers, and themselves. Through a weekly radio broadcast and special events, they raise community awareness about the issues surrounding long-term care.

Executive Director: Rev. Paul Falkowski

Since 1992, Desert Ministries has hosted several city and state-wide functions with the goal of creating intergenerational contacts during those events. In addition, they participate in community events by introducing nursing home residents as participants. Through their "GrandFriends" and "V.A.L.U.E" (Volunteers Assisting, Loving, and Uplifting Elders) programs, they create conduits for Christians to become involved in residents' lives.

Resources:
Desert Ministries offers several ministry resources at their website.

ELDERSOURCE BY DOBSON MINISTRIES

PO Box 1312
Greenville, SC 29602
Phone: 864-292-6592
Fax: 864-292-1227
Website: www.dobsonministries.org
Email: director@dobsonministries.org

The vision of ElderSource is to minister to the spiritual needs of infirmed seniors in eldercare facilities. *"They will still bear fruit in old age..." (Psalm 92:14).*

Their mission: As a free service to elder care facilities in the United Sates and Canada, ElderSource partners with facility activity directors and chaplains to develop effective volunteer-based one-to-one and group ministries, for edification and evangelization, featuring a "Resource Pack" of Christian-based audio/visual materials.

Executive Director: Stan Means

In 1979, The Dobson Tape Ministry was founded to help those in nursing homes who could no longer hold a Bible and read. With a small cassette player and the New Testament on tape, residents could once again experience God's Word.

Sensing the need to do more, a major change took place in 1996, which included adding the name "ElderSource". More materials were also added to their resource packet; including cassette tapes of older Gospel music, video tapes and devotional materials – all for the same price as in 1979 – free!

Resources:
ElderSource offers a free resource pack of these audio/visual materials to the Activity Director. Although the materials are free, the Activity Director must contact them for an application form.

FAITHFUL FRIENDS NURSING HOME MINISTRY

706 Crosswinds Dr.
West Palm Beach, Florida 33413
Phone: 561-434-4408
Fax: 561-965-1820
Website: www.faithfulfriends.org
Email: wass2@ix.netcom.com

The vision of Faithful Friends is to provide encouragement and support to nursing-home residents and volunteers who are sharing the love and message of Jesus in the nursing-home environment.

Their mission: Through regularly scheduled visits in area nursing homes, Faithful Friends spread the love and message of Jesus Christ through one-on-one visits and church services. They also support other interested groups and churches in Florida with training, multimedia ministry materials, and assistance in recruiting volunteers.

Ministry Director: Larry Wasserman

Faithful Friends maintains a very comprehensive web site on the Internet, which includes helps for how to get started in nursing home ministry, printable resources, information about other related organizations, links to most every nursing-home ministries websites, a bulletin board and their "Love Notes Newsletter". This site is regularly updated and expanded and includes a monthly drawing in which they give away valuable nursing-home ministry materials.

GOD CARES MINISTRY
33399 Walker Road Suite A
Avon Lake Ohio 44012
Phone & Fax 440-930-2173
Website: Godcaresministry.net
E-mail: Godcares@safe-t.net

The vision of God Cares Ministry is to provide quality Christ-centered spiritual care in long-term care centers that serve seniors.

Their mission is to recruit, train and support Christians who will establish a care team to adopt a long-term care center in their community. Volunteers are trained to assist the staff in meeting the spiritual needs of their residents by respectfully sharing God's love and Word. Though the primary focus of God Cares is Northeast Ohio, they continue to provide training and consultation throughout the USA and Canada.

Executive Director: Chaplain Bill Goodrich

Since 1994, God Cares Ministry has helped churches in Northeast Ohio develop over 125 care teams. Care Teams reach out in practical ways to individual residents and establish caring friendships that often result in helping them find peace, purpose, hope, and friendship with Jesus. Care teams are also trained to provide nondenominational church services, Hymn-sings and Bible studies for all interested.

Resources:
- God Cares Ministry has developed several training workshops to help churches throughout the USA and Canada establish effective ministries in long term care centers. Contact their office for information on hosting a workshop in your area.
- A bimonthly newsletter to encourage, instruct and inform nursing home missionaries. Subscriptions are free upon request.

LOVE YOUR NEIGHBOR MINISTRIES
PO Box 1886
Gresham, OR 97030
Phone & Fax: 503-491-1899
Website: www.lyn.org
Email: daveclyn@comcast.net

The vision of Love Your Neighbor is to build a broadening network of evangelical chaplains & volunteers, providing effective spiritual support through relationship building in long-term care.

Their mission is to assist the church through equipping and mobilizing God's people to reach out to lost, lonely & often forgotten people in the context of healthcare.

Executive Director: David Compton

Since 1975, Love Your Neighbor has been assisting the church in equipping people to reach out in compassion to those in hospitals, nursing homes and rehabilitation/care centers, retirement and assisted-care living, private homes through hospice and home health. Chaplains assist churches in volunteer training and oversight. They also focus on the needs of the extended families of those visited. LYN offers availability for ongoing grief support to those who have experienced the loss of loved ones.

Children also are encouraged to bring joy and hope to those in need. School, civic and church groups can be effective in reaching out to the elderly and infirm. Many of those visited have no family or friends and often have a few personal items at their bedside. Preparing and/or sponsoring a 'giftbag' filled with practical, personal items can fill a need and build a bridge of relationship with those visited. Businesses, foundations and churches are encouraged to partner with LYN in providing materials, groups and volunteers to help in meeting the need.

NURSING HOME MINISTRIES, INC.
PO Box 22246
Portland, OR 97269-2246
Phone: 503-771-4154
Fax: 503-771-0853
Website: www.nursinghomeministries.com
Email: nhminc@att.net

The Vision of Nursing Home Ministries is to reach out to adult care facilities in America with the love of our Lord.

Their mission is to recruit and train volunteer chaplains to serve wherever God opens the door.

Executive Director: Don DeBoer

Nursing Home Ministries was incorporated in Oregon in 1975. They have since become recognized throughout the nation for recruiting, training and commissioning chaplains to serve in adult-care facilities. NHM chaplains hold Bible classes and minister to all who would desire such service or ministry.

They also assist churches in making this ministry a vital part of their neighborhood ministry by training their members to visit nursing-home residents on a one-on-one basis. Through commissioned chaplains and volunteers, NHM is gaining access to and ministering in hundreds of adult-care facilities throughout the country. They recognize that there is much work to be done, and many facilities yet to reach. They welcome your prayers as they continue to reach new areas of service.

OUTREACH FOR CHRIST TO THE NURSING HOME MINISTRIES (OCNH MINISTRIES)

PO Box 226
Clarkston, MI 48347
Phone & Fax: 248-620-3231
Email: Ocnhlee@aol.com

The vision of OCNH is to reach out with the love of Christ to those who may not otherwise have the opportunity to hear the gospel.

Their mission is to develop, train and inspire volunteer teams to take the love and gospel of Jesus Christ to the residents of the nursing-care facilities, their families and staff. Their primary focus is Southeast Michigan.

Ministry Director: Chaplain Doug Lee

OCNH Ministries is a non-denominational faith-based ministry; They help assemble volunteer teams who visit a care facility for a regularly scheduled time of "Praise and Worship". Hymns are presented along with a reading from Scripture and a short message. Prayer requests are taken and prayed for. OCNH Ministries also offers a faith-based, nursing-home ministry "Training and Team-Building Workshop" in local churches. At these workshops, volunteers are equipped with the tools, information and training to prepare them for ministry in the nursing home.

SENIOR ADULT MINISTRIES AND SPECIAL PEOPLE

Phoenix First Assembly of God
13613 North Cave Creek Road
Phoenix, Arizona 85022
Phone: (602) 404-7415
Fax: 602-404-7026
Website: www.phoenixfirst.org
E-mail shenning@phoenixfirst.org

The vision of Senior Adult Ministries and Special People is to provide pastoral/spiritual care and services for all those living in long-term care centers or confined to private homes because of special needs.

Their mission is to provide services such as preaching, Bible studies, one-on-one visits, sing-a-longs, communion, memorials, weddings and advocacy resulting in Spiritual growth, nurturing and fellowship. They also maintain a fleet of specially equipped wheelchair-lift buses to provide transportation to church weekly and to other special events. SAMSP recruits and trains leaders, volunteers and chaplains in the how to's of Nursing Home Ministry.

Ministry Director: Pastor Sharon Henning

1 Corinthians 13:8, "Love Never Fails" is the motto of the SAMSP ministry. Since 1985, they have provided ministry to several thousand special-needs people in the Phoenix Metropolitan area. It is normal to see the entire front of their church filled with these special people, participating in the Sunday services.

Resources:

SAMSP has several teaching and training manuals, CD's, videos and cassette tapes for promoting, starting, enhancing and maintaining various kinds of ministries to people with special needs. See their web site.

SHARING JESUS MINISTRY

561 Montego Lane South
Ellenton, Florida 34222
Phone: 941-729-2062
Fax: 941-723-0021
Website: www.sharingjesusministry.org

The vision of Sharing JESUS Ministry is to share Jesus with those captive by age or circumstance, in nursing homes!

Their mission: In addition to personally ministering in nursing homes, Sharing Jesus Ministry helps other nursing home ministries create and maintain a 'base' website.

Ministry Director: Rev. Terrance R. Wilson

In 1996 as Terrance Wilson was searching the internet, and became painfully aware that he, as a Nursing Home Minister, was alone. He could not find any nursing home ministry websites! During the process of building his own site, still searching the internet for other nursing-home ministries, a few showed up in search. With hope and joy joined together with others to build a free service of providing a 'base' website design of one – ten pages for nursing-home ministries, with instructions on how to maintain their site.

THE SONSHINE SOCIETY
P.O. Box 327
Lynnwood, WA 98046
Phone: 425-353-4732
Website: www.sonshinesociety.org

The vision of The SonShine Society is to present a faithful Christian witness in nursing homes.

Their mission is to recruit, train and equip concerned lay-Christians to minister on a one-on-one basis or as part of a "Gospel Team" in a nursing home.

Ministry Director: Sharon Haakensen
Resource Contact: Patty Hawley

The SonShine Society was founded in 1973 by Herm Haakensen who saw the need for Christians to be challenged to provide a consistent and effective witness to people in care centers. Herm believed that age or physical impairment should not keep people from participating in the worship and instructional services of the Christian church. He therefore began to create materials to equip Christians for this vast harvest field. For Herm's last 30 years on earth, he was dedicated to the vision and mission of The SonShine Society.

SonShine continues to provide the nations largest supply of materials specifically designed for ministry in nursing homes (see resources on next page). People new to The SonShine Society are encouraged to contact them for a free Power Packet. This packet provides a basic training guide and samples of their ministry materials.

Sonshine Society Equipping Materials

- **SonShine Songs & Scriptures** – over 100 hymns and choruses and several Scripture portions for group ministry in Giant Print.
    * Also available are a piano/guitar leaders copy; sing-along cassette tapes and CD's, which match the songbook, word-for-word, (all pitched in a lower key).

- **Heaven, Heart and Home** – over 90 favorite old ballads, love songs, songs of our country, Christmas Carols and hymns in large print.
    * Also available are a piano/guitar leaders copy and sing-along cassette tapes, which match the songbook, word-for-word, (all pitched in a lower key).

- **Hope and Help** – Leaders resource with over 100 sermon illustrations and stories to which seniors can relate.

- **Strength and Peace** – A large-print Scriptural devotional that journeys through the old and new testament Bible.

- **Large print Scriptures** – Gospel of John and Paul's Epistles (KJV).

- **All the Days of My Life** – A step-by-step training guide to nursing home ministry.

- **Reaping the Harvest Training Video** -- A two-part video covering one-on-one and group ministry in nursing homes.

- **White unto Harvest Recruiting Video** – 17-minute video which presents the challenge of nursing home ministry. Includes 50 accompanying recruiting leaflets.

- **Giant-Print Tracts** – 4 and 8-page story tracts.

- **Giant-Print Greeting Cards** – Easter, Christmas, Birthday.

NURSING-HOME MINISTRY LEADER'S FELLOWSHIP

33399 Walker Road Suite A
Avon Lake Ohio 44012
Phone & Fax 440-930-2173

The Nursing Home Ministry Leader's Fellowship is a new fellowship of more than 20 nursing home ministry leaders from the USA and Canada. Most of them met for the first time in January 2003 to:

- establish a fellowship/communication that enables a clear understanding of each other's nursing home ministry.
- discover practical ways to support each other through closer relationships and prayer.
- consider ways to network in some common goals and practices.

Current contact person: Bill Goodrich

This first meeting was the beginning of a growing spirit of unity among Christ-centered Nursing Home Ministry Leaders who:

- have a deep love and concern for all people living in long-term care centers.
- have a ministry focus beyond their own church and are currently helping Christians throughout their region get involved with or develop a nursing home ministry.
- have a need and desire to support each other in prayer, communication and fellowship.
- have a willingness to work together, so that no nursing home resident is forgotten by the Christian church.

NHMLF plans to meet twice a year. If you are a nursing home ministry leader such as mentioned above, please give us a call to become connected.

OTHER HELPFUL RESOURCES

Devotionals and Bible study helps

The Upper Room – An interdenominational daily devotional (available in large print). USA: P.O. Box 37153, Boone, IA 50037. Canada: PO Box 3000 Toronto, ON M7Y 7A2.

Our Daily Bread – A daily devotional (available in large print). RBC Ministries. USA: PO Box 2222 Grand Rapids, MI 49501. Canada: Box 1622, Windsor, ON N9A 6Z7

Guideposts – Short true stories of hope and inspiration (available in large print). 39 Seminary Hill Road, Carmel, NY 10512.

Find it Fast in the Bible – By Ron Rhodes. A quick reference covering over 1000 Bible topics with more than 8000 Scripture references. (2000). Eugene, OR: Harvest House Publishers.

Full Circle: Spiritual Therapy for the Elderly – By Kevin H. Kirkland, & Howard McIlveen. Bible study outlines with suggested questions, songs and hymns on many different themes to use for ministering to people with dementia. Binghamton, NY: The Haworth Press.

Tears in God's Bottle: Reflections on Alzheimer's Caregiving – By Wayne Ewing. Poetic and practical reflections on caring for a wife with dementia. Written by a minister. (1999). Tucson, Arizona: WhiteStone Circle Press.

~~~

Inspirational reading for nursing home missionaries

Power of the Powerless – By Christopher De Vinck. A testimony to the power God demonstrates in the weakest vessels, in this case an immobile child who touched the lives of hundreds and taught them the true meaning of courage and perseverance. (1988). Pompton Plains, NJ: Zondervan.

Heart of Joy – By Mother Teresa A revealing of the heart of Mother Teresa's source of happiness, energy, and dedication, and the joy that comes from giving oneself to God and saying yes to whatever He asks. (1987). Ann Arbor, MI: Servant Books.

In My Own Words – By Mother Teresa (1989). Words that Mother Teresa shared with the poor, the dying, the hurting, and the skeptical. Liguori, MO: Liguori Publications.

My Journey into Alzheimer's Disease: A True Story – By Robert Davis. Helpful and insightful autobiography written by a minister who developed Alzheimer's disease at age fifty-three. (1989). Wheaton, IL: Tyndale House.

Alzheimer's: Caring for Your Loved One, Caring for Yourself – By Sharon Fish. Medical information and practical advice on how to cope with the demands of care giving and encouragement for handling tangled emotions and fears. (1996). Colorado Springs, CO: A Shaw Book/Water Brooke Press.

God Never Forgets: Faith, Hope and Alzheimer's Disease – By Donald K. McKim, Ed. Emphasis on how God can and still does relate to a person even if that person's ability to relate to God appears lost. (1997). Louisville, Kentucky: Westminster John Knox Press.

Counting on Kindness: The Dilemmas of Dependency – By Wendy Lustbader. Provides a touching overview and testimonies of both sides to care giving; from the caregivers perspective as well as the care receiver. (1991). New York: The Free Press.

Good Grief – By Granger Westberg. One of most helpful books visitors can give to people who have lost a loved one or are personally facing loss. Also available in large print. (1971). Philadelphia: Fortress Press.

Newsletters

Bits of Sonshine – By The Sonshine Society. Written to encourage Christian volunteers in nursing home ministry. Published five times each year. Lynwood, WA. ReJoyce Press, (See ministry profile on pages 252-253).

Care Tender – By Victoria McCarty, A monthly newsletter bringing encouraging words, inspiration and useful ideas to caregivers. Camano Island, WA: K-Bird Publications. Caretender.com

God Cares News – By God Cares Ministry. Written to encourage, instruct and inform nursing home missionaries. Published bi-monthly. Avon Lake, OH. (see ministry profile on page 246).

~~

Training and informational resources

A Song for Grandmother – By Dorothy Miller. A training guide for nursing home ministry, (A recruiting video is also available). (1990). Hemet, CA: Jeremiah Books.

A Handbook for Nursing Home Ministry – By Jerry and Darr Johnson.(1999). A guide to encourage and assist Christians in working together to meet the volunteer needs of every care facility in their geographical area. Norfolk, VA: Chapter and Verse, (see ministry profile on page 241).

Nursing Home Ministry: A Basic Training Guide – By Tom and Kaye DePinto. Provides basic yet detailed guidelines for those called to minister in nursing homes. (1991). Springfield, MO: General Council of the Assemblies of God, Chaplaincy Department.

Hands on Ministry. Helpful guidelines for chaplains and missionaries in health-care ministry. (1998). Texas Baptist

Volunteer Chaplaincy Training Manual. Dallas, TX Church Ministries: Baptist General Convention of Texas.

Large print and other-language Bibles

American Bible Society. 1865 Broadway, New York, NY 10023, americanbible.org

Christian Book Distributors. PO Box 7000 Peabody, MA 01961, Christianbook.com

International Bible Society. PO Box 35700 Colorado Springs, CO 80935, IBSDirect.com

Joni and Friends. P.O. Box 3333 Agoura Hills, CA 91376 joniandfriends.org (J.A.F. also has many great resources for ministering to those with disabilities.)

The Sonshine Society. PO Box 327 Lynnwood, WA 98046, sonshinesociety.org (See ministry profile on pages 252-253)

~~

Websites

Faithfulfriends.org The most extensive website we know of for nursing home ministry. Provides links to almost all other nursing home ministry websites. (See ministry profile on page 245)

Aahsa.org The American Association of Homes and Services for the Aging (AAHSA) represents not-for-profit organizations dedicated to providing high-quality health care, housing and services to the nation's elderly.

NursingHomeReports.com Provides an abundance of information related to the nursing home industry, including inspection reports on most nursing homes.

elderweb.com Provides a lot of up-to-date statistics and links regarding the nursing home industry.

ORDERING INFORMATION

This is our first printing of
NURSING HOME MINISTRY –
Where Hidden Treasures are Found.
We plan to run our second printing in mid 2004.
We are very interested in your thoughts regarding this book. If you have any comments or suggestions that might enhance our future printings, we would deeply appreciate you sending them to the address below.

For additional copies of this book contact:
God Cares Ministry
33399 Walker Rd., Suite A
Avon Lake, OH 44012
(440) 930-2173
Godcares@safe-t.net
Godcaresministry.net